HERBAL AID

by Edward Milo Millet

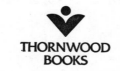

THORNWOOD BOOKS

1680 South Main
Springville, Utah 84663

Published by Thornwood Books
1680 S. Main
Springville, UT 84663

First Printing
May, 1980

ISBN 0-86588-014-X

Thornwood Books does not directly or indirectly dispense medical advise or prescribe the use of herbs as a form of treatment for sickness without medical approval.

Dedicated to all seekers of better health who believe in HERBS.

Table of Contents

Table of Contents

Introduction to HERBAL AID

A long time ago I saw that the real value in herbs is their use as foods and particularly that they would give valuable assistance for building strong body structures and facilitating wholesome systemal functions.

I discovered that herbs have a positive role in my quest for a healthier and happier lifestyle, and therefore they are necessary as regular additions to my daily diet and nutritional program.

Herbs have proven their worth to me and my family as foods by building our physical energies and vitality so that we do not have as many expenses for the usual physical ills and crises that plague many people these days. Because we feel better, the sunrise seems a little more beautiful, and the sun shines a little brighter for us each day. These special "resource foods" are effective not only as vitality aids and crisis preventives; herbs are equally helpful when body energies begin to fall and body systems fail to do their usual jobs.

Herbs are supportive of any systemal function that is acting up and becoming a problem! Herbs supply the necessary nutrients whereby any body system, part, or tissue can activate, cleanse, strengthen, and restore itself!

HERBAL AID is readily available from the immediate environment and also commercially in convenient, quality preparations. Anyone can take advantage of these special body foods and discover that herb power means life power!

Welcome to the wonderful world of herbs! Here you will meet many new friends, and nature itself will come alive to you as a warm and comforting surrounding. Like your fruit and vegetable garden, herbs (many of which are presently despised as mere "weeds") can help you physically when all other avenues seem to fail. Herbs are foods, enriched resources for giving the body an increased measure of strength, vigor, and vitality! Using herbs takes about as much skill as making a tossed salad. When you realize how simple it is to use herbs and how valuable they can be to your health, you will get tremendous enjoyment in improvising with various

1

herbs and herbal recipes to satisfy your own special needs.

Herbs are wonderfully simple, and simply wonderful! Feel free to experiment with them for your own health's sake. You will find some brief directions on page 4 to get you started.

Edward Milo Millet
Ethonobotanist and Herbalist

PART ONE
CHAPTER ONE

DIRECTIONS FOR GIVING EFFECTIVE HERBAL AID

Herbal aid is designed to give maximum understanding needed for the application of herbs, whatever a person's background and purposes. This book can be equally valuable to a concerned parent, an herb student, a nutritional consultant, or an herb practitioner.

A Word About Using HERBS vs. MEDICINES

Herbs are valuable resource foods for building body constitution and for fostering systemal vitality. This book is intended to increase knowledge and skills for using herbs as nutritional aids. Herbs give direct aid to the body processes so that they function more efficiently. Herbs also strengthen systemal structures, giving greater physical endurance and capability. Herbs are designed to supply an extra measure of the health-building materials that are vital for balancing the body's present critical needs.

Disease microorganisms, on the other hand, thrive where any unwholesome body condition persists. You can focus either on the failing systemal cause or on some resultant disease symptom. Herbs will help resolve the imbalance or deficiency so that you will experience a greater measure of health. Drug-medicines in reality only influence the symptom (i.e. microorganism activity). Herbs, therefore, are not synonymous with modern drug-medicines. There is a world of difference between using herbs and using drugs for health-related purposes. You can use herbs with absolute confidence because they are special foods. They are safe resource foods for building body constitution and systemal vitality. Drug-medicines have inherent dangers that signal considerable caution and risk. Regulated medicines and treatment of disease symptoms are the sole jurisdiction of licensed medical practitioners. Herbs and health, though, should be everybody's business! You can achieve more lasting results with herbs, which are the natural, non-toxic means to greater physical vigor and vitality. In the quest for a greater measure of health, you will find important guidelines to effective herb use in this book. By applying these simple principles and procedures, you can make responsible decisions for experiencing your own herb successes!

Giving yourself herbal aid is very simple

A few general rules-of-thumb for using either single herbs or herbal recipes (combinations) are:

1. When using aromatic herbs (herbs containing a fragrance or aroma) for body energizing:
   Take 2-4 capsules (single herb or herbal recipe) with ample warm water, or
   sip 1 cupful of warm herb tea (1 tea bag or 1 teaspoonful of powder steeped 10 - 15 minutes in hot water)
   three times daily before meals and also before bedtime.
2. When using bitter herbs (herbs containing bitter, distasteful properties) for body building and balancing:
   Take 1 - 3 capsules (single herb or herbal recipe) and 1 aromatic capsule (often capsicum) with ample cool water, or
   sip 1 cupful of cool herb tea (1 tea bag or ½ - 1 teaspoonful of powder simmered 10 - 20 minutes and allowed to cool
   three times daily with meals.
3. When using cosmetic herbs (herbs containing astringing/puckering or mucilaginous/slimy properties) for cleansing and beautifying:
   Take 2 - 3 astringent herb capsules (single herb or herbal recipe), and 1 aromatic capsule (often capsicum), with warm or cool water; or
   take 2 - 4 mucilaginous capsules (single herb or herbal recipe), and 1 aromatic capsule (often capsicum), with warm or cool water; or
   sip 1 cupful of herb tea (1 astringent tea bag, or 1 - 2

mucilage tea bags, or 1 teaspoonful of powder, simmered 10 - 20 minutes), used warm or cool
in the early morning on an empty stomach and between
meals.

These instructions will get you started in experiencing herbal successes. Remember that herbs are foods, enriched resources which should be used consistently in order to achieve
best results. As with other foods, there is no rigid standard
for preparing and using herbs. Feel free to experiment with
amounts (dosages) and frequency for taking herbs in order
to meet your own special physical needs.

Herbal aid correlates herb use with building body systems

Herbal aid will help you correlate the potential and value
of single herbs and herbal recipes (combinations) to the
needs and special requirements of particular body systems.
Herbs are foods and are nutrition oriented! Beginning with
the circulatory aids, which are energy activators, and in suc-
ceeding descriptions of each body system, herbal aid will—

(1) get you thinking positively about using herbs as "special foods" for strengthening body structures and activating
normal systemal functions;

(2) introduce the major single herbs that have proven historically successful for giving life power to particular body
systems;

(3) show you that these same single herbs can be blended
easily into effective herbal recipes (combinations). A number of herbal recipes for aiding each body system are listed
and can be studied to understand their compositions. These
selected herbal recipes historically have been highly prized for
their worth in supplying nutrient life for even the most difficult body conditions (NOTE: You don't need to be a qual-
ified herbalist or specialized chef in order to freely improvise
in using nature's foods for your own daily health-building
needs. As you gain experience in using herbal goods, you will

5

get amazing results, even from the beginning. As you grow in your ability to blend herbs and herbal recipes, you will achieve a greater measure of health!); and

(4) list those malfunctions that directly concern or otherwise affect each body system, define each common ailment or malfunction, and indicate which other body systems may be involved or affected.

Having this information about powerful herbal aids and understanding the body systems that herbs assist nutritionally, you should be able to use herbs selectively and effectively as "resource foods" for supplying nutrient aid to body systems, essential organs, and glands. Herbal aid is a proven means for gaining greater physical vitality! When your body receives adequate herbal aid, it becomes energized, cleansed, and balanced so that your physical movements have both "zest" and "zoom." Now isn't that what a quest for healthier and happier living requires?

How to use herbs as special resource foods for giving herbal aid

Herbs are beneficial, nutrition-plus foods that should be used the year-around, along with normal dietary intake. These herbal aids serve to—

(1) activate your body systems and structures to operate with greater energy;

(2) help body cleansing or purifying processes to eliminate more efficiently; and

(3) build and balance constitutional metabolism in all organs and tissues.

Follow this procedure of using herbal aids for normal health building

For normal health building, or preventive herbal aid, make sure that your daily program consists of selected supplements (either single herbs or preferably herbs in recipes or combinations) from each of the three nutritional categories indicated.

I. ENERGIZING

Use capsicum (cayenne), ginger, or other single herbs or herbal recipes (combinations), which are listed and described under the following systems: circulatory, nervous, respiratory, reproductive, urinary, sudoriferous, and digestive (for secretion activation).

II. BUILDING/BALANCING

Use alfalfa, dandelion, Irish moss, kelp, and other single herbs or herbal recipes (combinations) that are listed and described under the following systems: digestive, glandular, and intestinal.

III. CLEANSING/BEAUTIFYING

Use bayberry, white oak, myrrh, and other single herbs or herbal recipes (combinations) that are listed and described under the following systems: skin/membranous and muscular/skeletal. Also, give special cleansing herbal aid to the urinary, glandular (liver), and intestinal (lower bowel) operations.

Follow this procedure for using herbal aids in crisis health building

For crisis health building during unusual periods of body stress or distress, you can safely use herbal aids in mega-quantities—at least double or triple the normal recommended amounts. During physical struggles your body needs greater intake of special resource ingredients, so richly supplied in selected single herbs and which are mixed synergistically into effective herbal recipes or combinations. Generally, I prefer the results I get from using herbal recipes to the results I get from taking herbs singly. Herbal aids are especially welcome during periods of greater nutritional need, as their value is precious when you feel added power and life support going into faltering systems and structures.

7

Choose your herbal aids to fit your special crisis needs

You will get better health-building value by formulating your own weekly herbal aid program that is tailored to your special health-building needs in restoring particular body systems. In fashioning your herbal aid program, you should first emphasize herbal energizing and cleansing for 2 - 3 days, along with an alkalinizing procedure of using only selected mild foods and cleansing herbs or juices. That preparatory procedure should be followed by 3 - 4 days of herbal energizing and building/balancing, for giving essential strength and mineralization to your total body constitution and health building needs. During special times of crisis, you may select a megaquantity of herbal recipes (one or more combinations suited to your needs, and doubling or tripling the recommended use) or single herbs for cleansing and building the body. During times of crisis, the body craves the extra resource nutrient input. Added energy is needed to get circulation and nervous power into weak and sluggish tissues or parts. With an overload of body wastes and toxins that are irritating, obstructing, and weakening the entire body, as well as suppressing the problematic system or part, you can remove metabolic wastes more efficiently by applying the herbal aid emphasis which facilitates the purifying or cleansing processes. Last, you can rely on herbal aids for supplying your body with essential nutritional substances, particularly minerals that build the physical constitution and balance metabolic operations.

If your body is suffering only an acute stress condition, you can anticipate that herbal aid may give you rather quick results. If your body is undergoing a chronic distress state, you will have to work harder on your herbal aid program, repeatedly applying the alternating 2 - 3 day cleansing and 3 - 4 day building/balancing procedures over a much longer period of time (according to your own body's responses and needs). At these times the body must gradually regain its vitality within its own cyclic time, circumstances, and physical requirements. You can make that health-building process optimally possible by consistently supplying the body with regular and adequate herbal aid! The more difficult, lingering, and problematic distress conditions within any body system or part will require you to be extra patient with your herbal aid expectations. For these chronic distresses, you must be particularly persistent and consistent in supplying appropriate herbal materials for building and balancing the digestive, glandular, and intestinal systems.

An analytical systemal approach to more effective herbal aid

For giving restorative herbal aid to any irregularity within a weakening body system or part, you need to—

(1) support the system or part most affected and distressed, and

(2) strengthen the other systems that are either directly or indirectly involved.

For example, liver imbalance and irregularities can result in many complex disturbances within the skin, circulatory system, intestines, and elsewhere. Likewise, the liver is dependent on good digestive, circulatory, nervous, urinary, and other systemal operations.

The real secret for giving effective herbal aid

(1) Select the right herbal recipes (combinations) or single herbs that emphasize the nutritional resources most needed for resolving the pressing (stressing, distressing) failure conditions within the key system's faltering part(s).

(2) Give back-up assistance to other systems that are directly or indirectly involved in resolving that disturbed activity.

Again, giving herbal aid to needy body systems is simple and easy

(1) Select one or two herbal recipes (combinations) or major single herbs that are discussed under the system(s) requiring your special attention.

(2) Take the recommended amount for normal health building.

(3) Increase that to a megaquantity or take more often during crisis health building.

There is a unique philosophy associated with nutritional herbal aid

The following words and phrases are introduced for better defining herbal aid on a nutritional and resource food basis. Study them and review them periodically for a better understanding of herbal aid and its correct applications.

acute stress condition	an irregular function within the body that gives immediate discomfort, but may be resolved within a relatively short period of time
adequate herbal aid	each body system requires certain essential nutrients for maximum operation, and these must be supplied in sufficient quantity
body structures	the cells, tissues, and organs; the physical components of the body and its various systems
chronic distress state	the more disturbing, difficult, and lingering malfunctions that may involve structural impairments; requires more time, patience, and special care to resolve
cleansing juices	fruit and vegetable juices which can be used with selected herbs

	to help facilitate body eliminative processes
cyclic requirements	body processes are subject to gradual changes and also to cosmic influences, and these respond according to one's adherence to natural principles, or natural laws
crisis	a stressing or distressing condition that greatly taxes body energies and depletes vitalizing resources; often describes the lowest point in the life-power struggle within the body, after which considerable health betterment is realized
critical needs	each body system requires certain substances in an adequate supply in order to sustain its structures and functions
distress zone	the body system or part that is most affected or disordered, pained, or endangered, and thereby requires special nutritional attention
expertly-formulated (mixed)	correct application of herbal principles and successful experiences are necessary for gaining superior knowledge and skills (or expertise) with herbs and herbal aid
happiness	the state of radiant self-harm-

mony, expressed pleasure, and
purposive achievement

health
the state of optimum body dynamics, radiance, and wholeness.

herbal health building
herbs are resource foods that
support structural and functional vitality in the body

herbal aids
herbs have "plus ingredients"
that give added nutritive assistance to body structures and
functions

**herbal recipes
(combinations)**
herbs which are carefully selected according to their mutual
strengthening and reinforcing
(synergistic) activity in the
body; when blended together
and taken as a single herbal
good, these herbs manifest increased life-power as a nutritional team

normal recommended use
suggested herbal intake will
vary according to the type of
herb or herbal recipe, which is
usually indicated on the pack-
age or label of purchased herbs

life power
energies and capabilities for
zestful activity

life support
certain substances are essential
to sustain the body's structures and processes

12

malfunctions	weakening conditions in the body, resulting in irregularities to some body system(s) or part(s)
megaquantity	an increased consumption of selected herbal aids, needed to supply adequate supportive nutrition (especially during periods of stress or distress)
metabolic operation	total food processes in the body incidental to life, involving the peculiar building up and breaking down of nutrient substances, including all assimilation and elimination activities
mild foods	normal nutritional sources (mostly fruits and vegetables) that are more alkaline-forming in the body, and are neutralizing to excessive acid body conditions
mineralization	essential minerals (both major and trace) found in naturally-chelated compounds, which can be utilized in the body for achieving optimum strength and performance
mixed synergistically (herbal recipes)	combined so that the composite strengthening and mutually-reinforcing activites of the total substances are greater than any results from the individual parts; suggesting that

expertly formulated herbal recipes (combinations) can be expected to give superior and more effective health-building results

necessary nutrients

herbs supply various naturally-chelated compounds of minerals, vitamins, and other substances that are essential to maintaining the structures and functions of different body systems

normal dietary intake

the nutritive material (foods) that are regularly consumed for usual body metabolism and energy

nutrition-plus foods

herbs are supplementary "resource foods" that give added strength to body structures and tissues and activate and facilitate systemal operations

optimally possible

which will increase the systemal operations and capacities for greater constitutional potential

physical constitution

all supportive and operational activities in the body

problematic distress conditions

any systemal conditions suffering greatly reduced functional activity and possibly resulting in considerable structural discomfort or impairment

14

problematic system	a body system that is the seat or source of irregularity or malfunction, causing stress or distress to body functions and structures
proven historically successful	herbs have been the true body aids during many centuries, for giving extra power and life support to systemal needs and emergencies
restorative assistance	herbs contain substances that enable body systems to regain vitality and to operate efficiently
selected herbal recipes (combinations)	special mixtures of herbs that can supply enriched nutritional assistance to the particular needs of a body system or part
special resource foods	herbs contain enriched quantities of essential minerals and other needed substances for insuring body vitality
systemal functions	normal activities within a system that contribute to the larger body economy and actions
toxins	poisonous by-products of body metabolism which are very stressing and damaging to the body when not efficiently eliminated
vitality	the capacity for life power and

	the capability for expressing it; radiant animation
zest	an intense enjoyment and delightful relishing of life and its creative opportunities
zoom	powerful and sustained motion; energized momentum

Guidelines to herb power—from systemal weakness to body vigor!

The rightful role and use of herbs lies in health building, in supplying micronutrients, such as minerals, vitamins, and enzymes for restoring body structures and aiding various systemal operations.

In spite of an acknowledged positive reference that herbs are foods and that, historically, herbs have proven their value as body builders and systemal balancers, most persons today relate only to a negative reference in seeking some medicinal cure for apparent body ailments and diseases.

A disease, according to the natural reference, is merely a symptom, an indication of a deeper imbalance, and is the result of malfunction within the highly interrelated body systems. A disease, therefore, cannot be "cured" naturally in the popular sense of the word. Herbal aids can supply needed nutrition to failing system(s) and part(s), whereby these are energized, cleansed, and restored.

Herbs are more effectively used when they are considered as nutritional helps to body systems. When critical failing systems regain both structural and functional vitality, the more obvious symptoms (signs) of ailment will quickly disappear. For achieving real health, then, your focus on herbal aid should be positively oriented toward building (restoring and strengthening) body systems.

This guide to herbal aid is specially designed to direct your thoughts toward analyzing which body systems are related to and/or responsible for the weakened and ailing physical condition. Herbal aid helps you to supply immediate health-building support with selected herbal recipes or single herbs.

Once you have identified which body systems are involved in contributing to a particular weakness, then you can easily select the correct (most appropriate) herbal applications for achieving greater physical vitality. In fact, for herbal health-building successes it is as simple as "A-B-C!"

Round out your measure of health: give more balance to your lifestyle

The age-old adage, "As a man thinketh in his heart, so is he," is very important to your quest for achieving better physical well-being. Your deep purposes, heart's intents, and personal commitments do channel your physical energies and emotional states into certain patterns and determined ends. These attitudes and behaviors directly affect your body's nervous responses, circulatory functions, and especially the glandular secretions (including reproductive/sex hormone balances). Your physical substance is merely a vehicle and servant to your inner wishes, and it performs the patterns and plans that you commit your desires and resources to pursue. In brief, your well-being, vitality, and health depend chiefly on your total progress in bringing wholeness and balance into your lifestyle!

A person who is not in balance tends to fall into excesses. These excesses, in turn, foster more problems which hinder your desired self-enhancements and which bring you ultimate dissatisfacton. Your recognition of degenerating "side trips" or deceptions will keep you from reaping needless difficulties which result from following harmful dead-end programs. Your health will depend on the soundness of your whole life and your chosen lifestyle.

Let's list some of the holistic ingredients that you should consider and fashion into your lifestyle (mentioned here, but developed more fully in my other herbal health-building books):

SPIRITUAL well-being
MENTAL well-being
EMOTIONAL well-being
PHYSICAL well-being
SOCIAL well-being
ECONOMIC well-being
CULTURAL well-bing
CHARITABLE well-being
RECREATIONAL well-being

PART TWO

HERBAL AID FOR ENERGIZING/ INVIGORATING/REVITALIZING BODY SYSTMES

(using selected herbs with special aromatic properties)

Aromatic herbal aids are valuable resource foods for activating body energies, so that cellular metabolism and assimilation/elimination processes are significantly revitalized:

CIRCULATION is reinforced,
NERVES are recharged,
RESPIRATION is improved,
URINARY fluids are stabilized,
GENITAL/REPRODUCTIVE organs are sensitized,
SWEAT GLANDS are activated, and
DIGESTIVE secretions are stimulated.

Herbal aids to all these body systems have one characteristic in common: they are aromatics which contain important, volatile, fragrant substances that are called "essential oils." These body energizing herbal aids produce better results when they are taken in or with warm liquids. Aromatics are imperative for sustaining the body powers, and they should be available for immediate use during all emergency situations.

18

CHAPTER TWO

HERBAL AID FOR ENERGIZING THE CIRCULATORY OR CARDIOVASCULAR SYSTEM

Good circulation is essential for achieving optimum vitality

The circulatory system (comprising heart, arteries, and veins) is responsible for firing up your body's energy resources, so that warmth and power are felt in every system and part—including the extremities (arms and hands, legs and feet). Body stresses are greatly relieved with good circulation function because positive nutritional power is able to reach every living tissue, organ, and gland, while negative interferences from metabolic wastes and toxins are efficiently removed.

Good circulation will put noticeable vigor throughout the body's life-line. Circulation is greatly assisted by using selected aromatic herbs internally in the form of warm teas and herb capsules taken with warm water. Pay particular attention to the fact that your circulation needs ample water in order to facilitate its nutritional activities. Aromatic herbs help to boost and sustain body circulation by—

(1) increasing blood supply to the heart muscles so that they function with greater strength;

(2) assisting nervous responses in the heart so that nerve functions are regular and sustained; and

(3) feeding arterial and venous structures so that they retain elasticity and contractility, thereby avoiding problematic congestions and enabling an equalized nutritional flow into all body parts.

Externally, these aromatic herbs are valuable circulation aids—herbal fomentations, compresses, liniments, oils, baths, vapor baths, washes, footbaths, and so forth (introduced in my HELP YOURSELF! textbook, Course 1).

Besides using selected herbal aids for strengthening circulation, you will want to participate in hard physical labor or vigorous exercise (sports, jogging, hiking, swimming, etc.); drink ample water; use body massage; slant-board exercise, grass or sand walking; maintain good posture; build emotional stability, and so forth. A body that is always fatigued and lethargic really is a poor vehicle for getting you where you want to go. You can get much better physical mileage, at energy savings, if you commit yourself to apply some of the natural means that are available for you to achieve better body care.

Major characteristics of single herbs which supply circulatory aid

CAPSICUM or CAYENNE fruit
Capsicum annuum, C. frutescens

Considered the strongest and most persisting circulatory activator known; its pungent oil makes a burning sensation on the stomach membrane, but it has a deserved reputation as a powerful herb for soothing and restoring skin/membranous malfunctions

GINGER root
Zingiber officinale

A valuable herb for strengthening venous circulation; it also activates digestion, relieves putrefactions (gases and flatulence) and spasms, and is an excellent genital/reproductive aid

SIBERIAN GINSENG root
Eleutherococcus senticosus

A truly great constitutional restorer for circulatory (blood activator and balancer), nervous (sensitizes functional responses and coordination, energizer), digestive, glandular (increased endurance, enzyme catalyst, emotional balancer), genital (hormone), respiratory, skin/membranous, urinary, and intestinal systems

GARLIC bulb
Allium sativum

Powerful circulation restorative, high in sulphur content
and organic penicillin, useful
liver activator, effective herbal
aid to nervous, respiratory,
and digestive systems

HAWTHORN berry
Crataegus oxyacanthus

Powerful herbal aid for the
circulation, with specific nutritional resource ingredients for
building heart tone

ROSEMARY leaves
Rosmarinus officinalis

Especially invigorating to circulation, an important ingre-
dient for skin/membranous
beauty care; also a cleanser/
builder of nervous, genital/
reproductive, respiratory, and
urinary systems

WATERCRESS herb
Nasturtium officinale

Valuable circulation activator
and blood builder (rich in organic mineral compounds),
also glandular (liver), urinary,
and other systems

Basic herbal recipes (combinations) for supplying circulatory aid

_____ garlic bulb, capsicum fruit,
(clove flowers)

_____ capsicum fruit, Siberian ginseng root, gotu kola herb,
(prickly ash bark, wild ginger
root)

_____ hawthorn berry, capsicum fruit, garlic bulb, (blessed thistle herb, motherwort herb, wild ginger root)

_____ garlic bulb, capsicum fruit, parsley root, ginger root, Siberian ginseng root, golden seal root, (hyssop herb, thyme herb)

_____ garlic bulb, rose hips, rosemary leaves, parsley herb, watercress herb, (thyme herb, eucalyptus leaves)

Problems and malfunctions involving the circulatory system

acidosis

Acid/alkaline imbalance in the blood or body tissues, in which acids increase and alkalinity decreases.
DIGESTIVE, GLANDULAR, URINARY, MEMBRANOUS

Adams-Stokes syndrome

Consciousness affected by decrease of blood to the brain, usually caused by heart problems.
CIRCULATORY, NERVOUS, GLANDULAR, MUSCULAR

alkalosis

Excessive alkaline condition of the body.
DIGESTIVE, GLANDULAR, CIRCULATORY

22

amyocardia, heart weakness Weakness of heart muscle.
MUSCULAR, CIRCULA-
TORY, NERVOUS, GLAN-
DULAR

anemia Reduction of red blood cells
in circulation.
GLANDULAR, CIRCULA-
TORY, DIGESTIVE

aneurysm Abnormal local dilation of
blood vessel due to weakness
in a vessel wall.
MUSCULAR, CIRCULA-
TORY, GLANDULAR

angina pectoris Sharp pain and pressure on the
heart due to some structural
impairment of the heart.
MUSCULAR, NERVOUS,
CIRCULATORY, GLAN-
DULAR

angitis, angiitis Inflammation of blood or lym-
phatic vessels.
MEMBRANOUS, GLANDU-
LAR, CIRCULATORY

aortitis Inflammation of the aorta.
MEMBRANOUS, GLANDU-
LAR, CIRCULATORY, URI-
NARY

arteriolosclerosis Loss of elasticity and con-
tracility in walls of the small
arteries.
MUSCULAR, CIRCULA-
TORY, GLANDULAR

23

arteriosclerosis	Thickening and hardening of blood vessel walls. MUSCULAR, GLANDULAR, CIRCULATORY
arteritis	Inflammation of an artery. MEMBRANOUS, GLANDULAR, CIRCULATORY
bleeding, hemorrhage	Process of emitting blood. CIRCULATORY, MEMBRANOUS/MUSCULAR, GLANDULAR
blood (purity) problems	GLANDULAR, URINARY, INTESTINAL
cardiovascular problems	CIRCULATORY, NERVOUS, MUSCULAR, GLANDULAR, URINARY, INTESTINAL
chills	Attack of shivering, accompanied by a sensation of coldness and paleness of skin. CIRCULATORY, NERVOUS, GLANDULAR
circulation problems	CIRCULATORY, GLANDULAR, DIGESTIVE, MUSCULAR
congestion	Excessive amount of blood or fluid in an organ or tissue. CIRCULATORY, GLANDULAR, URINARY, MUSCULAR, NERVOUS

coronary/heart problems	CIRCULATORY, NERVOUS, MUSCULAR, GLANDULAR
embolism	Obstruction of a blood vessel by a blood clot or foreign substance. CIRCULATORY, GLANDULAR
energy problems	CIRCULATORY, NERVOUS, GLANDULAR, URINARY, INTESTINAL, DIGESTIVE
exhaustion	Loss of vital powers, extreme fatigue. CIRCULATORY, NERVOUS, GLANDULAR, DIGESTIVE
fatigue	Tiredness or weariness from overexertion and reduced energy level. CIRCULATORY, NERVOUS, GLANDULAR, DIGESTIVE
first aid, herbal	CIRCULATORY, NERVOUS, MUSCULAR, GLANDULAR
heart problems	CIRCULATORY, NERVOUS, MUSCULAR, GLANDULAR
heart failure	Heart malfunction resulting in an inability to maintain adequate blood circulation. CIRCULATORY, NERVOUS, MUSCULAR, GLANDULAR
heat cramps	Sharp painful spasms of voluntary muscles after hard

work in a hot environment, due to insufficient fluids and sodium loss.
CIRCULATORY, <u>NERVOUS</u>, <u>MUSCULAR</u>, GLANDULAR

heat exhaustion

Heat prostration or extreme weakness and functional collapse, from profuse sweating and loss of body salts through physical exertion in a hot environment.
CIRCULATORY, <u>NERVOUS</u>, <u>MUSCULAR</u>, URINARY, DIGESTIVE, GLANDULAR

heatstroke, sunstroke

Dangerous reaction to heat exposure, resulting in cessation of sweating, high body temperature, and functional collapse.

hemophilia

Blood clotting disorder, resulting in abnormal bleeding tendency (prone to males).
CIRCULATORY, <u>GLANDULAR</u>, MEMBRANOUS/ MUSCULAR

high blood pressure

Hypertension of circulating blood on arterial structures.
CIRCULATORY, <u>MUSCULAR/MEMBRANOUS</u>, <u>GLANDULAR</u>, NERVOUS

hypertension

Excessive tension or blood pressure in circulatory vessels— see "high blood pressure."

lactation problems	CIRCULATORY, MEM-BRANOUS/MUSCULAR, GLANDULAR
lethargy	A condition of reduced functional activity, sluggishness. CIRCULATORY, NERVOUS, GLANDULAR/URINARY/INTESTINAL
leukemia	Abnormal leukocyte increase in tissues (particularly the blood-forming organs) and in circulation. GLANDULAR, CIRCULATORY, DIGESTIVE
mastitis	Breast inflammation, usually with infection. CIRCULATORY, MEM-BRANOUS/MUSCULAR, GLANDULAR
milk deficiency	See "lactation problems."
mononucleosis	Abnormal increase in the blood's content of mononuclear leukocytes, particularly affecting the spleen and lymph nodes. GLANDULAR, CIRCULATORY, URINARY
myocarditis	Inflammation of heart muscular tissue. MUSCULAR, GLANDULAR, CIRCULATORY

night sweat(s)
Profuse sweating at night during sleep, indicates body weakness.
<u>CIRCULATORY</u>, <u>NERVOUS</u>, <u>GLANDULAR</u>, DIGESTIVE

nursing problems
<u>CIRCULATORY</u>, <u>GLANDULAR</u>, MEMBRANOUS/ MUSCULAR, DIGESTIVE, NERVOUS

obstruction
Abnormal blocking or clogging of a structure or channel, hindering its normal function.
<u>CIRCULATORY</u>, <u>GLANDULAR</u>, MEMBRANOUS/ MUSCULAR, URINARY, INTESTINAL

pallor
Lack of color or paleness of the skin.
<u>CIRCULATORY</u>, NERVOUS, SKIN, GLANDULAR, DIGESTIVE

palpitation
Rapid abnormal throbbing or fluttering of the heart.
<u>NERVOUS</u>, <u>CIRCULATORY</u>, MUSCULAR, GLANDULAR, DIGESTIVE, INTESTINAL

phlebitis
Inflammation of a vein.
<u>CIRCULATORY</u>, <u>MEMBRANOUS/MUSCULAR</u>, GLANDULAR, URINARY

prostration

Complete loss of strength, resulting in mental and physical exhaustion.
CIRCULATORY, NERVOUS, GLANDULAR, DIGESTIVE

Raynaud's disease

Abnormal spasm in blood vessels of extremities, especialy when responding to cold temperatures, resulting in swelling and pain (rare in males).
CIRCULATORY, NERVOUS, GLANDULAR

tachycardia

Abnormal rapid heart action.
NERVOUS, CIRCULATORY, GLANDULAR, MUSCULAR, DIGESTIVE, INTESTINAL

temperature problems

CIRCULATORY, MEMBRANOUS/SKIN, NERVOUS, GLANDULAR, URINARY

thrombosis

Formation or presence of a blood clot within a blood vessel.
CIRCULATORY, MEMBRANOUS, GLANDULAR, DIGESTIVE

varicose veins

Enlarged and twisted veins.
CIRCULATORY, MEMBRANOUS/MUSCULAR, GLANDULAR/URINARY

vascular problems   CIRCULATORY, MEM-
                                 BRANOUS, NERVOUS,
                                 GLANDULAR/URINARY

vein/venous problems   CIRCULATORY, MEM-
                                 BRANOUS, NERVOUS,
                                 GLANDULAR/URINARY

vitality, strength problems CIRCULATORY, NERVOUS,
                                 GLANDULAR, DIGESTIVE,
                                 URINARY/INTESTINAL

CHAPTER THREE
HERBAL AID FOR ENERGIZING THE NERVOUS OR NEUROLOGIC SYSTEM

Good nerves increase body sensitivity and zest

The nervous system (comprising brain, spinal cord, and nerves) is responsible for regulating and coordinating all the body's energy resources. Its control centers direct the power functions and expressive capabilities for all body organs and systems—eyes, ears, skin, joints, muscles, and taste, smell, touch.

Body stresses are often translated into nervousness, altered emotions, mental irregularities, and functional disturbances—all of which are favorably influenced when appropriate nerve nutrients are supplied. Good nervous tone and balance will give zest to your body's expressive dynamics. Nerves are greatly assisted by using selected aromatic herbs internally in the form of warm teas and herb capsules taken with warm water. Aromatic herbs help to stabilize and recharge body nerves by—

(1) feeding neurons and related tissues directly with requisite supportive nutrition;

(2) activating circulation so that body assimilation is improved and waste products are more efficiently removed;

(3) stabilizing brain functions so that mental and emotional states are positively oriented;

(4) stimulating needed secretions so that glandular activities are balanced;

(5) supplying oxygen for giving strength and vitality to nerves; and

(6) coordinating all body parts into harmonious and healthful activity.

Externally, these aromatic herbs are valuable nerve aids as herbal fomentations, compresses, liniments, oils, lotions, baths, vapor baths, washes, footbaths, and the like (introduced in my HELP YOURSELF! textbook, Course 1).

Besides using selected herbal aids for nerves, you will want to commit yourself to an active and purposeful program of planned work, complete relaxation, regular exercise, outdoor recreation, fresh air and sunshine, creative fulfillment, heartwarming sociability, charitable service, and so on. A sensitized body that also possesses reason and purpose is capable of harmonizing its energy functions and of directing its available creative resources toward achieving any worthwhile goal that its heart may desire!

Major characteristics of single herbs which supply nerve aid

LADY'S SLIPPER root *Cypripedium pubescens*	One of nature's most powerful and effective nervous restoratives, often referred to as "American valerian"
LOBELIA herb *Lobelia inflata*	Considered to be one of nature's greatest restoratives for the entire body, but more specifically it is recommended for the severe stress or distress crisis conditions (in combination with other herbs); beneficial for nervous, glandular, respiratory, membranous/skin, genital/reproductive, muscular, and intestinal systems; especially useful for aiding any difficult and obstructive systemal conditions
SCULLCAP herb *Scuterllaria lateriflora*	A powerful nervous tonic and relaxant, especially building to the central nervous system
VALERIAN root *Valeriana officinalis*	An especially strong and reliable, quieting and soothing nerve aid for building and restoring all power-related conditions; also promotes digestive and intestinal secretions

32

BLACK COHOSH root
Cimiciguga racemosa

A powerful nerve aid that beneficially influences glandular (liver, lymphatics), circulatory, genital/reproductive (female hormone), and urinary functions

SIBERIAN GINSENG root
Eleutherococcus senticosus

A truly great constitutional restorer for nervous (sensitizes functional responses and coordination, energizer), glandular (enzyme activator, emotional balancer), circulatory (blood activator and tension balancer), genital, respiratory, urinary, intestinal, and other systems

HO SHOU-WU or **EUROPEAN SOLOMON'S SEAL** root
Polygonatum multiflorum, Convallaria multifloria

Excellent nerve aid for restorative purposes; excellent influence on digestive, glandular, nervous, skin/membranous, muscular, genital, respiratory, urinary, and intestinal systems— a general systemal builder

WOOD BETONY leaves
Betonica officinalis, Pedicularis canadensis

Excellent nerve aid for brain and general nervous malfunctions, also a blood cleanser by activating liver and spleen functions

MISTLETOE leaves
Viscum album

A valued nerve aid for any nervous debility or excitement (for heart, brain, nerves)

ST. JOHNSWORT tops
Hypericum perforatum

Power restorer for respiratory, nervous, glandular, genital, urinary, intestinal, skin/membranous, and muscular systems

GOTU KOLA herb
Hydrocotyle asiatica

Valued nerve activator and tonic; specific respiratory cleanser/restorer; glandular strengthener and blood purifier

WILD LETTUCE herb
Lactuca virosa
and species

Important nerve balancer and calmative; reproductive tonic; glandular activator

HOPS flowers
Humulus lupulus

Activating and balancing nerve tonic; circulation and heart strengthener; respiratory restorer; digestive aid; urinary activator, glandular (liver, gallbladder) cleanser/restorer

Basic herbal recipes (combinations) for supplying nerve aid

_____ valerian root, wild lettuce leaves, capsicum fruit, (clove flowers, lobelia herb, wild ginger root)

_____ black cohosh root, capsicum fruit, valerian root, mistletoe herb, ginger root, St. Johnswort herb, hops flowers, wood betony herb, (wild ginger root, passion flower herb, lady's slipper root)

_____ valerian root, scullcap herb, hops flowers, (wood betony herb, lady's slipper root)

_____ blessed thistle herb, black cohosh root, scullcap herb, pleurisy root, (lobelia herb, echinacea root, St. Johnswort herb)

_____ blessed thistle herb, periwinkle herb, capsicum fruit, ginger root, lobelia herb, blue vervain herb, (mistletoe herb, rosemary leaves, garden sage leaves)

_____ black cohosh root, capsicum fruit, valerian root, mistletoe herb, lady's slipper root, lobelia herb, scullcap herb, hops flowers, wood betony herb, (passion flower herb, clove flowers, prickly ash bark, ginger root)

_____ safflower oil, oil of wintergreen, menthol, camphor, (oil of wormwood, oil of myrrh)

Problems and malfunctions involving the nervous system

brain problems   NERVOUS, CIRCULATORY, GLANDULAR

cephalalgia, headache   Pain in the head, symptom of various disorders
GLANDULAR/INTESTINAL/ URINARY, NERVOUS, CIRCULATORY

cerebral problems   NERVOUS, CIRCULATORY, GLANDULAR

claustrophobia   Fear of being confined in a closed space.
NERVOUS, GLANDULAR

coma   State of profound unconsciousness or mental sluggishness.
CIRCULATORY, NERVOUS, GLANDULAR

concussion   Jarring injury (particularly to brain), or loss of function due to hard blow or collision with an object.
NERVOUS, CIRCULATORY, GLANDULAR

consciousness problems   CIRCULATORY, NERVOUS, GLANDULAR

deafness   Partial or complete loss of hearing.
NERVOUS, CIRCULATORY, GLANDULAR

delirium   Excited and confused mental state, manifesting disorienta-

tion and incoherence.
CIRCULATORY, NERVOUS,
GLANDULAR

delirium tremens

Violent physical/mental disorder involving hallucinations
and physical trembling, caused
by excessive use of alchoholic
beverages.
NERVOUS, CIRCULATORY,
GLANDULAR, MUSCULAR,
DIGESTIVE

dementia

State of mental deterioration.
NERVOUS, CIRCULATORY,
GLANDULAR

depression

Mental state of sadness, self-
depreciation, and low spirit.
CIRCULATORY, NERVOUS,
GLANDULAR

dizziness, vertigo

Mental state of confusion, gid-
diness, or whirling sensation
with a tendency to fall.
CIRCULATORY, NERVOUS,
GLANDULAR

encephalitis, phrenitis

Inflammation of the brain.
MEMBRANOUS/MUSCU-
LAR, CIRCULATORY,
NERVOUS, GLANDULAR,
URINARY

epilepsy

Neurological attack disturbing central nervous and brain
functions, especially affecting

motor, sensory, psychic and consciousness functions, and may be accompanied by convulsions.
NERVOUS, CIRCULATORY, GLANDULAR, DIGESTIVE

equilibrium problems

NERVOUS, GLANDULAR, CIRCULATORY

fear

Anxiety and emotional reaction to a threat or danger.
NERVOUS, GLANDULAR, CIRCULATORY

fit, convulsion

Sudden attack with violent emotion or action.
NERVOUS, CIRCULATORY, GLANDULAR

frustration

State of energy discontrol from an unsatisfactory obstacle or thwarting of intended acts and purposes.
NERVOUS, CIRCULATORY, GLANDULAR

hallucination

Nervous disorder resulting in false sensory perceptions and illusions that are confused as reality.
NERVOUS, GLANDULAR, CIRCULATORY

headache

Diffuse pain in the head.
NERVOUS, CIRCULATORY, GLANDULAR/URINARY/ INTESTINAL

hiccough, hiccup	Inspiratory cough caused by spasmodic closure of the glottis. NERVOUS, MEMBRANOUS
hydrocephalus	Abnormal increase of cerebro-spinal fluid within brain cavities. CIRCULATORY, MUSCULAR, NERVOUS, GLANDULAR
hyperactive, hyperactivity	Excessive functional activity. NERVOUS, GLANDULAR
hysteria	Abnormal mental and emotional imbalance, with high susceptibility to extreme excitability. NERVOUS, GLANDULAR, CIRCULATORY, DIGESTIVE
insanity	Severe mental disorder with hallucinatory tendencies and inability to distinguish right from wrong. NERVOUS, CIRCULATORY, GLANDULAR, URINARY/ INTESTINAL
insomnia	Abnormal wakefulness and inability to sleep. NERVOUS, GLANDULAR, DIGESTIVE
mania	Excessive mental excitement, with delusions of grandeur,

and so on.
NERVOUS, CIRCULATORY,
GLANDULAR

melancolia

Mental state of extreme depression, loss of will power, indifference, and the like.
NERVOUS, CIRCULATORY,
GLANDULAR

memory problems

NERVOUS, CIRCULATORY,
GLANDULAR

meningitis

Inflammation of membranes
of the spinal cord or brain.
NERVOUS, MEMBRANOUS,
CIRCULATORY, GLANDU-
LAR, URINARY/INTESTI-
NAL

mental problems/disease

NERVOUS, CIRCULATORY,
GLANDULAR, DIGESTIVE

migraine

Sudden, severe, and reoccuring
attack of headache, with visual
disorders and gastrointestinal
disturbances.
NERVOUS, CIRCULATORY,
GLANDULAR, DIGESTIVE,
URINARY/INTESTINAL

multiple sclerosis

Partial or complete paralysis
and jerking muscle tremors
progressive degeneration of
central nervous system due to
patches of hardened tissue in
the brain or spinal cord.

NERVOUS, GLANDULAR,
CIRCULATORY, MUSCU-
LAR, DIGESTIVE

myelitis

Inflammation of the spinal
cord or bone marrow.
GLANDULAR, SKELETAL,
NERVOUS, CIRCULATORY

narcotism

Addiction to narcotics or drugs
used to depress the central nervous system for pain relief, to
induce sleep, create false eu-
phoria, and so forth.
NERVOUS, GLANDULAR,
CIRCULATORY, DIGES-
TIVE

negatism, negativism

Skeptical mental attitude or
contrary behavior.
NERVOUS, GLANDULAR,
CIRCULATORY, DIGES-
TIVE

nerve/nervous problems

NERVOUS, CIRCULATORY,
GLANDULAR, DIGES-
TIVE, URINARY/INTESTI-
NAL

nervousness

Uneasiness or unrest associated
with nervous excitability or
irritation.
NERVOUS, CIRCULATORY,
GLANDULAR

neuralgia

Severe, sharp pain radiating
along the course of a nerve.

NERVOUS, CIRCULATORY,
MUSCULAR, GLANDU-
LAR, URINARY/INTESTI-
NAL

neuritis

Inflammation of a nerve or
nerves, usually associated with
pain, sensory disturbances, and
reflex degenerations.
NERVOUS, CIRCULATORY,
GLANDULAR, URINARY/
INTESTINAL

neurosis

Functional nervous disorder,
resulting from mental and
emotional conflicts.
NERVOUS, GLANDULAR,
CIRCULATORY, DIGES-
TIVE

nicotine poisoning,
tobacco habit

Effects from smoking or chew-
ing tobacco.
NERVOUS, GLANDULAR,
DIGESTIVE, RESPIRA-
TORY, CIRCULATORY

nightmare

Frightening dream accompanied
by a sense of suffocation.
NERVOUS, CIRCULATORY,
GLANDULAR

nightwalking

State of walking about while
sleeping.
NERVOUS, GLANDULAR,
CIRCULATORY

otalgia, earache

Pain in the ear.
NERVOUS, CIRCULATORY,
MEMBRANOUS, GLANDU-

obsession

Abnormal preoccupation with an idea or emotion, damaging when it develops into an all-compelling neurosis.
NERVOUS, GLANDULAR

pain

Unpleasant, discomforting, or distressing sensation due to some body disorder or injury, often associated with inflammation.
NERVOUS, MUSCULAR, CIRCULATORY, GLANDU-DULAR/URINARY/INTES-TINAL

paralysis

Nervous degeneratin resulting in partial or complete loss of function (especially voluntary motion or sensation).
NERVOUS, MUSCULAR, CIRCULATORY, GLANDU-LAR, DIGESTIVE

paranoia

Excessive persecution complex with delusions of self-grandeur.
NERVOUS, GLANDULAR

personality problems

NERVOUS, GLANDULAR, CIRCULATORY, DIGES-TIVE

perversion

Deviation or abuse of a normal function or behavior.
NERVOUS, GLANDULAR DIGESTIVE

pessimism

Negative and gloomy mental condition.
NERVOUS, GLANDULAR, CIRCULATORY, DIGESTIVE

phobia

Any abnormal fear.
NERVOUS, GLANDULAR, CIRCULATORY, DIGESTIVE

poliomyelitis

Inflammation of the gray matter of the spinal cord, resulting in motor paralysis and muscular degeneration.
NERVOUS, CIRCULATORY, GLANDUALR, MUSCULAR

psychoneurosis

Nervous and glandular malfunction due to unresolved conflicts in the subconciousness, resulting in decreased ability to perform responsibilities.
NERVOUS, GLANDULAR, CIRCULATORY, DIGESTIVE

psychosis

Severe mental disorder of personality disintegraton and loss of contact with reality, resulting in delusions and hallucinations.
NERVOUS, GLANDULAR, CIRCULATORY, DIGESTIVE

psychosomatic disorder

Disorder due to mental con-

flicts, resulting in emotional disturbances and other physical symptoms.
NERVOUS, GLANDULAR CIRCULATORY, DIGESTIVE

rabies, hydrophobia

Infectious nervous disease attacking the central nervous system, transmitted through a rabid animal bite (usually a dog).
NERVOUS, GLANDULAR MUSCULAR, CIRCULATORY

reflex problems

NERVOUS, MUSCULAR, CIRCULATORY, GLANDULAR

relaxation problems

NERVOUS, CIRCULATORY, MUSCULAR, GLANDULAR

schizophrenia

Mental disorder resulting in loss of contact with environment, accompanied by personality disintegration.
NERVOUS, GLANDULAR, CIRCULATORY, DIGESTIVE, URINARY, INTESTINAL

sciatica

Severe pain along the course of the sciatic nerve, felt at the back of the thigh and going down the inside of the leg.
NERVOUS, CIRCULATORY, MUSCULAR, GLANDULAR

senility	Degenerative mental disorder, incidental to physical weakness in old age. <u>NERVOUS</u>, <u>CIRCULATORY</u>, <u>GLANDULAR</u>, DIGESTIVE
sense/sensory problems	<u>NERVOUS</u>, <u>CIRCULATORY</u>, <u>GLANDULAR</u>, SKIN/MEMBRANOUS
sensual	Abnormally indulgent of appetites, or preoccupied with sensory gratification. <u>GLANDULAR</u>, <u>NERVOUS</u>, <u>GENITAL/REPRODUCTIVE</u>, DIGESTIVE, CIRCULATORY
shock	Violent disturbance to mental and emotional equilibrium, resulting in circulatory disorder and decrease in oxygen to tissues. <u>NERVOUS</u>, <u>CIRCULATORY</u>, GLANDULAR
smelling problems	<u>NERVOUS</u>, <u>MEMBRANOUS</u>, CIRCULATORY, GLANDULAR
sleepwalking, somnabulism	Sleeping state in which motor action is performed, but not remembered. <u>NERVOUS</u>, <u>GLANDULAR</u>
spinal cord problems	<u>NERVOUS</u>, <u>CIRCULATORY</u>, <u>GLANDULAR</u>

stress

Physical or mental tension which alters the existing systemal balances.
NERVOUS, GLANDULAR, CIRCULATORY

stupor

Extreme suppression of sense or feeling resulting in apathy and tiredness.
NERVOUS, CIRCULATORY, GLANDULAR

stuttering

Spasmodic repetition of a syllable in speech.
NERVOUS, MUSCULAR, GLANDULAR

suicidal tendency

State of mental depression or insanity that could result in self-murder.
NERVOUS, GLANDULAR, CIRCULATORY, DIGESTIVE

taste problems

NERVOUS, GLANDULAR, CIRCULATORY, MEMBRANOUS

tremor

An involuntary, convulsive quivering movement.
NERVOUS, MUSCULAR, GLANDULAR, CIRCULATORY

von Recklinghausen's disease

Multiple tumors of the nervous sheath.
GLANDULAR, NERVOUS, MUSCULAR

CHAPTER FOUR

HERBAL AID FOR ENERGIZING THE RESPIRATORY OR BRONCHO-PULMONARY SYSTEM

Good respiratory function delivers the breath of life to every body part

The respiratory system (comprising the nose, larynx, pharynx, trachea, bronchi, pleura, and lungs) is responsible for intensifying the body's energy capabilities and enabling an integration of power into general body metabolism. The respiratory activities make possible the breath or spark of life (oxygenation) for all other systems and parts. Any respiratory disturbances impaired gas exchanges, membranous obstructions, foreign substances, and circulatory pollutions, will result in lowered body vitality, increased metabolic disorders, tissue degenerations, and a sharp reduction to all systemal performances. Good respiratory tone will quicken every other physical response and enhance the body's structural capabilities.

Respiration (principally by the lungs) is greatly assisted by using selected aromatic herbs internally in the form of warm teas and herb capsules taken with warm water. Aromatic herbs reinforce and regulate body respiration by—

(1) strengthening the critical nervous responses so that the breath operation is sustained;

(2) improving arterial and venous circulation so that the blood flows properly and bathes the tissues adequately;

(3) aiding membranous activity so that gas exchanges (oxygen, carbon dioxide) occur efficiently;

(4) activating tissue secretions so that air is sufficiently moisturized and sensitive surfaces are protected; and

(5) stimulating glandular and urinary functions so that metabolic by-products and other impurities are rapidly extracted from the life-bearing bloodline and are thereby kept from disturbing and polluting its important operations. Externally, these aromatic herbs are valuable respiratory aids as

48

herbal vapors, footbaths, fomentations, compresses, oils, liniments, vapor baths, washes, and so on (which are introduced in the Help Yourself! textbook, Course 1).

Besides using selected herbal aids for the lungs, you will want to exercise actively (for better oxygenation), rest adequately (for metabolic restitution), acquire purifying living habits and a positive living/working environment (for avoiding unnecessary destructive pollutants), form good nutritional habits (to build blood composition and capacity), and foster a wholesome and creative lifestyle (in order to promote nervous balance and glandular harmony). A body that receives intensification of its energy resources is capable of greater creative purpose, faster responsive action, and more sustained worthwhile direction!

Major characteristics of single herbs which supply respiratory aid

COMFREY root
Symphytum officinale

Powerful and esteemed lung restorative with high calcium content, soothing and healing properties

MULLEIN leaves
Verbascum thapsus

Special respiratory affinity; pain-reliever and restorer for lingering stress conditions (especially mucous and serious membranes); softening and soothing to skin/membranes

THYME herb
Thymus vulgaris

Valuable respiratory tonic and relaxant (with cleansing, antiseptic, disinfectant, and healing properties); excellent digestive and nervous aid; also aids urinary, genital, glandular, intestinal, and skin/membranous systems

YARROW herb
Achillea millefolium

Excellent circulation activator, respiratory cleanser and tissue strengthener, sweat gland and urinary activator, blood purifier

RED CLOVER tops
Trifolium pratense

Efficient respiratory activator/ cleanser/tonic, blood purifier, nervous balancer, skin and tissue restorer

ROSE hips
Rosa canina

Circulation strengthener, respiratory aid (high vitamin C); activates membranous and urinary secretions

CAPSICUM or **CAYENNE** fruit
Capsicum annuum,
C. frutescens

Considered the strongest and most persisting circulatory activator known, activates membranous secretions and restores tissues, strengthens respiratory and urinary functions

LOBELIA herb
Lobelia inflata

Powerful nervous and glandular balancer; activates respiratory secretions; removes obstructions and congestions

GARDEN SAGE leaves
Salvia officinalis

Excellent aid to circulation and nerves, respiratory cleanser and tissue restorer, reproductive balancer, glandular and urinary activator, digestive and intestinal builder

Basic herbal recipes (combinations) for supplying respiratory aid

_____ fenugreek seeds, thyme herb, (myrrh gum)

_____ comfrey root, marshmallow root, mullein leaves, slippery elm bark, lobelia herb, (thyme herb, eucalyptus leaves)

_____ rose hips, chamomile flowers, slippery elm bark, yarrow herb, capsicum fruit, golden seal root, myrrh gum, peppermint leaves, (garden) sage leaves, lemongrass herb, (eucalyptus leaves, St. Johnswort herb)

_____ comfrey root, mashmallow root, lobelia herb, chickweed herb, mullein leaves, (eucalyptus leaves, pleurisy root root)

_____ ginger root, capsicum fruit, golden seal root, licorice root, (myrrh gum, echinacea root)

_____ lobelia herb, mullein leaves, (echinacea root, blue flag root)

_____ comfrey root, fenugreek seeds, (eucalyptus leaves)

_____ bayberry rootbark, ginger root, white pine bark, capsicum fruit, cloves flowers, (prickly ash bark, hemlock spruce tree bark)

_____ garlic bulb, rose hips, rosemary leaves, parsley herb, watercress herb, (thyme herb, eucalyptus leaves)

Problems and malfunctions involving the respiratory system

angina, quinsy

Attack of choking or suffocation, because of a disorder of the pharynx or throat.
NERVOUS, RESPIRATORY, GLANDULAR, MEMBRANOUS, CIRCULATORY

anoxia

Oxygen deficiency.
GLANDULAR, RESPIRATORY, CIRCULATORY

anthracosis, black lung

Discoloration of lungs by overexposure to coal dust and silica.
RESPIRATORY, GLANDULAR, CIRCULATORY

anthrax

Infectious animal disease contracted by contact with animal parts.
RESPIRATORY, GLANDULAR, MUSCULAR, URINARY/INTESTINAL

asthma

Spasmodic pain and difficult breathing caused by bronchial hypersensitivity or membranous disorder.
RESPIRATORY, NERVOUS, CIRCULATORY, MEMBRANOUS, GLANDULAR

breathing problems RESPIRATORY, NERVOUS, CIRCULATORY, GLANDULAR

bronchial problems RESPIRATORY, NERVOUS, CIRCULATORY, GLANDULAR

bronchitis Inflammation of bronchial mucous membrane. RESPIRATORY, MEMBRANOUS, CIRCULATORY, NERVOUS, GLANDULAR

chest problems RESPIRATORY, CIRCULATORY, MEMBRANOUS, GLANDULAR

choking Obtructing or interfering with breathing or circulation of blood to brain. CIRCULATORY, RESPIRATORY, NERVOUS, GLANDULAR

cold, coryza Catarrhal inflammation of respiratory mucous membranes. RESPIRATORY, MEMBRANOUS, CIRCULATORY, GLANDULAR

cough Forceful expulsion of air from the lungs, often caused by inflammation of the respiratory

tract.
RESPIRATORY/CIRCU-
LATORY, MEMBRANOUS,
NERVOUS, GLANDULAR

croup, laryngitis

Inflammation and spasm of larynx, usually with difficult and suffocative breathing, also a dry and hoarse cough.
MEMBRANOUS, NERVOUS, CIRCULATORY, RESPIRA-TORY, GLANDULAR

diphtheria

Bacterial formation of a false membrane on a mucous mem-brane surface, sometimes a complication causing a dan-gerous obstruction of the air passage.
CIRCULATORY, GLANDU-LAR, MEMBRANOUS, NER-VOUS

drowning

Blockage of respiratory func-tion by a laryngeal spasm, or water (fluids) in the lungs.
CIRCULATORY, NERVOUS, RESPIRATORY, GLANDU-LAR

dyspnea

Labored or difficult breathing.
CIRCULATORY, NERVOUS, RESPIRATORY, GLANDU-LAR

emphysema

Distension and loss of elasti-city of lung tissues, usually

54

from inhaling gases (such as smoking), with resultant functional impairment.
RESPIRATORY, MUSCULAR, CIRCULATORY, GLANDULAR

empyema

Pus in a body cavity, such as the pleural cavity, usually from lung infection.
RESPIRATORY/CIRCULATORY, MUSCULAR, GLANDULAR

flu, influenza, grippe

Contagious viral infection of the respiratory tract, usually accompanied by fever, cold, coughing, chills, inflammation, prostration, etc., and lasts 2-7 days.
RESPIRATORY, SUDORIFEROUS, CIRCULATORY, NERVOUS, GLANDULAR/ URINARY/INTESTINAL

halitosis, bad breath

Offensive odor on breath, usually from stomach disorders.
DIGESTIVE, CIRCULATORY, MEMBRANOUS, GLANDULAR

hay fever

Sensitive allergic response (especially to pollens, dust) of mucous membranes of the nose and upper respiratory passages, with catarrh and inflammation

of the eyes.
GLANDULAR, RESPIRA-TORY/CIRCULATORY
MEMBRANOUS

hoarseness

Inflammation causing a rough quality to the voice.
MEMBRANOUS, CIRCU-LATORY, GLANDULAR

lung problems

RESPIRATORY, MEMBRA-NOUS, CIRCULATORY, NERVOUS, GLANDULAR

mountain fever, soroch

Condition of subnormal oxy-genization of the blood occur-ring when persons ascend to higher altitudes (over 10,000 feet), resulting in various cir-culatory, nervous, and other disorders.
CIRCULATORY, RESPIRA-TORY, NERVOUS, GLAN-DULAR

pectoral problems

RESPIRATORY, CIRCULA-TORY, NERVOUS, MEM-BRANOUS, GLANDULAR/ URINARY/INTESTINAL

pertusis, whooping cough

Infectious catarrhal disorder resulting in a convulsive spas-modic cough, ending in a whooping or crowing inspira-tion of breath.
RESPIRATORY/CIRCULA-TORY, NERVOUS, GLAN-DULAR

pharyngitis	Inflammation of the pharynx or throat. MEMBRANOUS, CIRCU-LATORY, NERVOUS, GLANDUALR
phthisis	Degenerative and wasting pulmonary disorder. RESPIRATORY, GLANDU-LAR, CIRCULATORY, NERVOUS, URINARY/IN-TESTINAL
pleurisy	Inflammation of the pleura or serious membrane covering the lung. MEMBRANOUS, RESPIRA-TORY/CIRCULATORY, GLANDULAR
pneumonia	Inflammation of the lung. RESPIRATORY/CIRCULA-TORY, MEMBRANOUS/MUSCULAR, NERVOUS, GLANDULAR/URINARY/INTESTINAL
psittacosis	Infectious disease of birds transmitted to man, resulting in respiratory inflammation, diarrhea and wasting. RESPIRATORY, MEMBRA-NOUS, GLANDULAR, CIR-CULATORY, DIGESTIVE, INTESTINAL
pulmonary problems	RESPIRATORY, MEMBRA-

NOUS, CIRCULATORY, NERVOUS, GLANDULAR

respiratory/respiration problems

RESPIRATORY, NERVOUS, CIRCULATORY, GLANDULAR

sore throat

Painful inflammation of the tonsils and throat.
MEMBRANOUS, CIRCULATORY, GLANDULAR, NERVOUS, DIGESTIVE

speech problems

MEMBRANOUS, NERVOUS, CIRCULATORY, GLANDULAR, DIGESTIVE

throat problems

RESPIRATORY/CIRCULATORY, MEMBRANOUS, GLANDULAR, DIGESTIVE

tonsil problems

GLANDULAR, MEMBRANOUS, CIRCULATORY

tonsillitis

Inflammation of the tonsils.
GLANDULAR, CIRCULATORY, MEMBRANOUS

tuberculosis

Infectious, inflammatory disorder resulting in respiratory degeneration.
RESPIRATORY/CIRCULATORY, MEMBRANOUS, GLANDULAR

voice/vocal problems

MEMBRANOUS, CIRCULATORY, NERVOUS, GLANDULAR

CHAPTER FIVE

HERBAL AID FOR ENERGIZING THE URINARY OR RENAL SYSTEM

Good urinary function will keep the circulatory lifeline cleansed and balanced

The urinary system (comprising the kidneys, bladder, ureters, and urethra) is responsible for extracting waste substances from the blood, for regulating its water content, and for filtering the electrolyte substances or blood salts (especially sodium, potassium, calcium, and magnesium). The urinary activities are enhanced by a strong and effective circulation (blood pressure), the volume of water intake, dietary selection, nervous responsiveness, and so forth. As the kidneys are the chief eliminative agent for the body, several negative factors can contribute to urinary difficulties: excessive waste acids in circulation, polluting foreign substances taken into the body (drugs, alcohol, synthetics, and the like), indiscrete and irregular living habits, reabsorption of fecal putrefactions, circulation malfunctions, sweat gland suppression, and the like. Also, any urinary disturbances will increase body stress, decrease circulatory efficiency, reduce the effectiveness of systemal cleansing, and result in energy loss and physical sluggishness. Good urinary activity will keep the circulation channels cleansed of unwanted burdens and balance its alkaline/acid content.

Urinary performance (principally the kidneys) is greatly assisted by using selected aromatic herbs internally in the form of warm teas and herb capsules taken with sufficient warm water. Aromatic herbs reinforce and regulate urinary activity by—

(1) sustaining arterial and venous circulation so that blood velocity and osmotic pressure are adequate;

(2) regulating the nerve supply so that urinary functions are coordinated;

(3) supplying electrolytes (minerals) so that the acid/alkaline content of the blood is balanced;

(4) activating membranous secretions for lubricating sensitive surfaces and facilitating the unwanted waste expulsion;

(5) controlling water levels in the body so that general metabolism is aided and sustained; and

(6) maintaining sensitive tissues that are the important filters to body lifeline fluids.

Externally, these aromatic herbs are valuable urinary aids as herbal baths, fomentations, sitzbaths, douches, footbaths, oils, vapors, and so on.

Besides using selected herbal aids for the urinary system, drink ample water, eat properly, be physically active, rest sufficiently, discard intemperant habits, and balance your lifestyle. A body with life fluids that are both clean and capable will have no energy shortage, and body systems will be supplied with ample food resources for achieving any desired and worthwhile goal!

Major characteristics of single herbs which supply urinary aid

JUNIPER berries
Juniperus communis

Great urinary invigorator and herbal aid; counteracts and cleanses systemal toxicity; also strengthens nerves, genital/reproductive, muscular, and other systems

UVA URSI or **BEARBERRY** leaves
Arctostaphylos uva-ursi

A specific for all acute and chronic urinary distresses; also a valuable genital/reproductive restorer; cleansing tannic and gallic acids, counteracts acidity; antiseptic and disinfectant

PARSLEY leaves
Petroselinum sativum

One of the best kidney and liver herbs for restoring chronic distress conditions

BUCHU leaves
Barosma crenata

Another urinary specific for distress conditions activating/ cleansing/protective tonic; influences circulatory, respiratory, glandular, and membranous systems

CORN silk
Zea mays

One of the most effective herbs for distressed urinary conditions; counteracts acidity and soothes degenerating surfaces

HORSETAIL or **SHAVEGRASS** herb
Equisetum arvense, E. hyemale

Powerful membrane and tissue cleanser, with high silicon and calcium content, antiseptic and disinfectant; relieves and firms degenerating tissue surfaces, powerfully cleansing due to tannin

GRAVEL ROOT, QUEEN OF THE MEADOW root
Eupatorium purpureum

Powerful urinary activator/ cleanser/tonic; nervous restorer; strengthens membranes and tissues; reproductive and glandular cleanser/balancer

DANDELION root
Taraxacum officianale

Valued systemal alkalinizer; reliable urinary cleanser/tonic; glandular activator (liver, gallbladder, spleen, pancreas), blood builder (rich in organic mineral compounds), digestive restorer

YARROW herb
Achillea millefolium

Excellent circulation activator, blood purifier, and systemal cleanser; special influence on sweat glands and urinary system; restores and balances uterine functions

Basic herbal recipes (combinations) for supplying urinary aid

_____ juniper berries, parsley herb, uva ursi leaves, dandelion root, chamomile flowers, (couchgrass root, cleavers herb)

_____ golden seal root, juniper berries, uva ursi leaves, parsley herb, ginger root, marshmallow root, lobelia herb, (couchgrass root, gravel plant leaves)

_____ juniper berries, uva ursi leaves, licorice root, capsicum fruit, mullein leaves, golden seal root, (prickly ash bark, eucalyptus leaves, elecampane root)

_____ juniper berries, golden seal root, capsicum fruit, parsley herb, ginger root, Siberian ginseng root, uva ursi leaves, queen of the meadow (gravel root) root, marshmallow root, (prickly ash bark, myrrh gum, sarsaparilla root)

_____ golden seal root, juniper berries, uva ursi leaves, huckleberry leaves, mullein leaves, comfrey root, yarrow herb, garlic bulb, capsicum fruit, dandelion root, marshmallow root, buchu leaves, bistort root, licorice root, (prickly ash bark, blue flag root, elecampane root)

Problems and malfunctions involving the urinary system

albuminuria

Excessive protein in urine, usually signals renal impairment.
URINARY, GLANDULAR, DIGESTIVE

anuresis

Urine suppression or insufficient kidney secretion.
URINARY, CIRCULATORY, NERVOUS, GLANDULAR

bedwetting, enuresis

Incontinence or involuntary urination, either partial (nocturnal) or complete.
URINARY, NERVOUS, GLANDULAR

bladder problems

URINARY, MEMBRANOUS, CIRCULATORY, GLANDULAR, DIGESTIVE

Bright's Disease, nephritis

Kidney disease, associated with albuminaria and dropsy.
URINARY, MEMBRANOUS, GLANDULAR

calculus, calculi

Abnormal concretion or stone in the urinary tract.
URINARY, MEMBRANOUS,

GLANDULAR, NERVOUS, DIGESTIVE

colicystitis
Bladder inflammation from infection.
URINARY, MEMBRANOUS, GLANDULAR

cystitis
Bladder inflammation.
URINARY, MEMBRANOUS, GLANDULAR

dehydration
Excess reduction of body fluids.
URINARY, CIRCULATORY, GLANDULAR

dropsy, hydrops, anascara
Abnormal fluid accumulation in body tissues and cavities.
URINARY, GLANDULAR, MEMBRANOUS, CIRCULATORY

dysuria
Painful or difficult urination.
URINARY, NERVOUS, CIRCULATORY, MUSCULAR

edema
Localized condition of excessive fluids in body tissues due to circulatory, lymphatic, urinary, or other disorders.
CIRCULATORY, URINARY, GLANDULAR, MEMBRANOUS, DIGESTIVE

enuresis, incontinence
Involuntary urination or inability to retain urine, partial

64

(nocturnal or diurnal) or complete.

URINARY, NERVOUS, MUSCULAR, GLANDULAR

gravel, stone

Concretions of crystals from the kidneys.

URINARY, MEMBRANOUS, GLANDULAR, CIRCULATORY, NERVOUS, DIGESTIVE

hematuria

Blood in urine.

URINARY, MEMBRANOUS, GLANDULAR

incontinence

Inability to retain or control urination or defecation.

NERVOUS, MUSCULAR, URINARY, GLANDULAR

kidney problems

URINARY, CIRCULATORY, MEMBRANOUS, NERVOUS, GLANDULAR

lithiasis

Formation of calculi and concretions, stones and gravel.

URINARY, MEMBRANOUS, GLANDULAR, CIRCULATORY

nephritis

Kidney inflammation.

URINARY, MUSCULAR, CIRCULATORY, GLANDULAR, NERVOUS

pyelitis

Inflammation of a kidney pel-

vis.
URINARY, MUSCULAR, GLANDULAR, CIRCULA-TORY

retention, ischuria

Inability to urinate.
URINARY, NERVOUS, MEMBRANOUS, CIRCULA-TORY, GLANDULAR

strangury

Painful and spasmodic urina-tion.
NERVOUS, URINARY, MUS-CULAR, GLANDULAR

uremia

General toxic condition result-ing from deficient urinary/kid-ney function.
URINARY, CIRCULATORY, NERVOUS, GLANDULAR

ureteritis

Inflamed ureters.
MEMBRANOUS, URINARY, CIRCULATORY

urinary/urine problems

URINARY, MEMBRANOUS, CIRCULATORY, NERVOUS, DIGESTIVE

CHAPTER SIX

HERBAL AID FOR ENERGIZING THE GENITAL OR REPRODUCTIVE SYSTEM

Superior genital function is the fount of creative fertility for the entire body

The genital system (comprising ovaries, fallopian tubes, uterus, vagina, and so on, for females; and testes, seminal ducts, penis, spermatic cord, prostate glands, and so on, for males) is responsible for giving greater fertility and expressive power to the body, so that energies can become transformed and refined to greater potential. These important organs are involved with catalyzing physical development, facilitating creative expression, and sensitizing other organs and glands into more refined capability.

Balanced genital activity will greatly enhance your creative capacities and opportunities. Genital vitality is greatly assisted by using selected aromatic herbs internally in the form of warm teas and herb capsules taken with warm water. Aromatic herbs will supply added power to enhance genital fertility, by—

(1) improving circulation so that systemal nutrition is maintained;

(2) normalizing nervous responses so that power responses are optimal;

(3) balancing glandular functions so that secretions are sufficient and sustained; and

(4) activating more vigor and coordinating harmonious functions in all body parts.

Externally, these aromatic herbs are valuable genital aids as herbal douches, sitzbaths, baths, oils, lotions, fomentations, and footbaths (which are introduced in my Help Yourself! texbook, Course 1.) The herbal sitzbath is particularly valuable for aiding pelvic/abdominal operations—circulation is strongly sustained, muscles are strengthened, membranes are cleansed and activated.

Besides using selected herbal aids for the genitalia, you will want to commit yourself to a lifestyle which balances your total body energies—mental, emotional, physical, and spiritual. The genital/reproductive system is instrumental in bringing forth the flowering of body potentials, and its special care will multiply your creative opportunities!

Major characteristics of single herbs which supply genital/ reproductive aid

BLACK COHOSH root
Cimicifuga racemosa

Powerful nervous activator/ balancer; genital strengthener (female hormone); glandular (liver, lymphatics) and urinary restorer

BLESSED THISTLE or **HOLY THISTLE** herb
Cnicus benedictus, Carbenia benedicta

Valued activator/tonic for the reproductive system; also energizer for circulation (and heart); strengthens brain and nerves; aids digestion and balances the liver

• **RED RASPBERRY** leaves
Rubus idaeus, R. strigosus

A favorite gentle genital stimulative tonic, especially for pregnancy, high in iron and organic compounds for blood-building

SIBERIAN GINSENG root
Eleutherococcus senticosus

Great constitutional restorer and functional balancer; energizer to genital, nervous, circulatory, glandular, and digestive systems

SAW PALMETTO berries
Serenoa serrulata, Sabal palmetto

Effective constitutional and genital restorer; rich in minerals and hormones; effective for digestive, glandular, urinary, skin/membranous and other systems

SARSAPARILLA root
Smilax officinalis
and related species

Powerful glandular and genital balancer and restorer, rich in minerals; effective for reproductive (male and female hormones), skin/membranous, muscular/skeletal, and urinary systems

FALSE UNICORN root
Chamaelirium luteum

Powerful stimulative tonic to genital structures and functions; strengthening to membranes; gives urinary and digestive aid

PENNYROYAL herb
Mentha pulegium

Very reliable uterine activator/cleanser/tonic; purifies and removes obstructions; nervous strengthener/balancer/calmative; muscular restorer

BLUE COHOSH root
Caulophyllum thalictroides

Important Indian herb for childbirth, strengthening uterine muscles and activating nervous energy; circulatory stimulator and tension balancer

● **SQUAW VINE** herb
Mitchella repens

Another highly esteemed Indian herb for reproductive malfuntions of all types; helpful for activating urinary and strengthening membrane systems

CRAMP BARK bark
Viburnum opulus var. americanum

One of the best herbs for reproductive distresses during pregnancy, especially for relieving pains, spasms, and other nervous malfunctions

DAMIANA leaves
Turnera aphrodisiaca, T. diffusa

Valued as a genital rejuvenator and tonic; strengthens nervous energies; activates circulation

LICORICE root
Glycyrrhiza glabra

Valued glandular balancer; cleanses and strengthens tissues; aids digestive, respiratory, urinary, and intestinal systems

Basic herbal recipes (combinations) for supplying genital/ reproductive aid

_____ black cohosh root, false unicorn root, squaw vine herb, blessed thistle herb, lobelia herb, pennyroyal herb, red raspberry leaves, (wild ginger root, bayberry rootbark, motherwort herb)

_____ black cohosh root, squaw vine herb, lobelia herb, pennyroyal herb, red raspberry leaves, (false unicorn root, wild ginger root, bayberry rootbark)

_____ black cohosh root, licorice root, false unicorn root, Siberian ginseng root, sarsaparilla root, squaw vine herb, blessed thistle herb, (prickly ash bark, capsicum fruit, wild ginger root)

_____ golden seal root, capsicum fruit, false unicorn root, ginger root, uva ursi leaves, cramp bark, squaw vine herb, blessed thistle herb, red raspberry leaves, (myrrh gum, yellow dock root, dandelion root)

_____ golden seal root, red raspberry leaves, black cohosh root, queen of the meadow herb, marsh-mallow root, blessed thistle herb, lobelia herb, capsicum fruit, ginger root, (clove flowers, prickly ash bark, yellow dock root)

_____ Siberian ginseng root, echina-cea root, saw palmetto berries, gotu kola herb, damiana leaves, sarsaparilla root, periwinkle herb, garlic bulb, capsicum fruit, chickweed herb, (Virginia snakeroot root, prickly ash bark, blue flag root)

_____ ginger root, capsicum fruit, golden seal root, licorice root, (myrrh gum, prickly ash bark)

_____ black cohosh root, licorice root, kelp plant, gotu kola herb, golden seal root, capsicum fruit, ginger root, lobelia herb, (myrrh gum, prickly ash bark, blue flag root)

_____ comfrey root, golden seal root, yellow dock root, squaw vine herb, marshmallow root, chickweed herb, mullein leaves, slippery elm bark, (myrrh gum, prickly ash bark, clove flowers, bayberry rootbark)

_____ comfrey root, grapevine, Ho shou wu/European Solomon seal root, ginger root, alfalfa herb, blessed thistle herb, red raspberry leaves, peppermint herb, golden seal root, (blue cohosh root, dandelion root)

Problems and malfunctions involving the genital/reproductive system

abortion

Premature termination of pregnancy and expulsion of the fetus (usually 20-28th week of gestation).
REPRODUCTIVE, MUSCULAR, GLANDULAR, NERVOUS, CIRCULATORY, DIGESTIVE

amenorrhea

Suppressed or lack of menstruation.
REPRODUCTIVE, CIRCULATORY, NERVOUS, GLANDULAR, DIGESTIVE

anaphrodisia	Lack of or diminished sexual capability. REPRODUCTIVE, NERVOUS, GLANDULAR, CIRCULATORY, MUSCULAR, DIGESTIVE
androphobia	Abnormal fear of the male sex. REPRODUCTIVE, GLANDULAR, NERVOUS
aphrodisia	Excess sexual passion. REPRODUCTIVE, GLANDULAR, NERVOUS, CIRCULATORY
breast problems	CIRCULATORY, GLANDULAR, MEMBRANOUS, NERVOUS
childbirth problems	REPRODUCTIVE, NERVOUS, CIRCULATORY, GLANDULAR, MUSCULAR
chlorosis	A form of iron-deficiency anemia. GLANDULAR, DIGESTIVE, CIRCULATORY
delivery assistance (pregnancy)	REPRODUCTIVE, CIRCULATORY, NERVOUS, MUSCULAR, GLANDULAR
douche aids	MEMBRANOUS/MUSCULAR, GLANDULAR, CIRCULATORY

dysmenorrhea Painful menstruation. CIRCULATORY/REPRODUCTIVE, NERVOUS, GLANDULAR

embryo development DIGESTIVE, GLANDULAR, CIRCULATORY, REPRODUCTIVE, MUSCULAR, NERVOUS

erection problems REPRODUCTIVE, NERVOUS, GLANDULAR, CIRCULATORY

estrogen deficiency REPRODUCTIVE, GLANDULAR, DIGESTIVE

female problems REPRODUCTIVE, GLANDULAR, DIGESTIVE, CIRCULATORY, NERVOUS

feminism Abnormal dominance of female characteristics by the male. REPRODUCTIVE, GLANDULAR, DIGESTIVE, CIRCULATORY, NERVOUS

frigidity Abnormal sexual indifference, especially in a woman, indicating hormone and glandular disturbance. REPRODUCTIVE, GLANDULAR, CIRCULATORY, NERVOUS, DIGESTIVE

genital problems REPRODUCTIVE, GLANDULAR, CIRCULATORY,

74

	NERVOUS, DIGESTIVE, URINARY/INTESTINAL
gonorrhea	Contagious, infectious, inflammatory social disease of the genital mucous membrane. GLANDULAR, MEMBRANOUS, REPRODUCTIVE, URINARY, CIRCULATORY, NERVOUS
hot flashes	Abnormal reaction during menopause, result of glandular imbalance, in which skin capillaries of head, neck, and chest dilate, causing flushing, sweating, and a hot suffocating sensation. GLANDUALR, CIRCULATORY, NERVOUS, REPRODUCTIVE, DIGESTIVE
impotence, sterility	Sexual weakness of male, incapability for intercourse or reproduction. REPRODUCTIVE, GLANDULAR, CIRCULATORY, NERVOUS, DIGESTIVE
labor, childbith, delivery, parturition	Process of expelling the fetus from the uterus. REPRODUCTIVE, NERVOUS, CIRCULATORY, MUSCULAR, GLANDULAR
leukorrhea	White or yellowish vaginal discharge resulting from inflam-

mation or congestion of the mucos membrane.
MEMBRANOUS, GLANDULAR, REPRODUCTIVE, CIRCULATORY, URINARY

masturbation
Abnormal self-stimulation of sex organs, usually to orgasm.
REPRODUCTIVE, GLANDULAR, CIRCULATORY, NERVOUS

menopause, climacteric
Period of menstrual cessation, usually at 45-55 years of age, affecting circulatory, nervous, and glandular functions.
CIRCULATORY, GLANDULAR, NERVOUS, REPRODUCTIVE, DIGESTIVE

menorrhagia
Excessive menstrual bleeding.
CIRCULATORY, MEMBRANOUS, GLANDULAR

menstruation problems
REPRODUCTIVE, CIRCULATORY, NERVOUS, GLANDULAR, URINARY, DIGESTIVE

metrorrhagia
Spotty, extra-menstrual bleeding.
MUSCULAR, REPRODUCTIVE, CIRCULATORY, GLANDULAR

miscarriage
Premature expulsion of the fetus in pregnancy, between the 3rd and 7th months, usually

due to body weakness.

REPRODUCTIVE, MUSCU-LAR, CIRULATORY, NER-VOUS, GLANDULAR, DI-GESTIVE

morning sickness, nausea

Nausea and vomiting during the first few months of preg-nancy, particularly manifest upon rising in the morning.

DIGESTIVE, NERVOUS, GLANDULAR, CIRCULA-TORY, REPRODUCTIVE

nymphomania

Excessive abnormal sexual de-sire by a female.

REPRODUCTIVE, NER-VOUS, GLANDULAR, CIR-CULATORY, DIGESTIVE, URINARY/INTESTINAL

orchitis

Testicle inflammation.

REPRODUCTIVE, MEM-BRANOUS, GLANDULAR, CIRCULATORY, NERVOUS

orgasm difficulty

Emotional state occurring at the climax of sexual inter-course (female) or upon ejacu-lation of semen (male).

REPRODUCTIVE, NER-VOUS, GLANDULAR, CIR-CULATORY, DIGESTIVE

ovary/ovarian problems

REPRODUCTIVE, GLAN-DULAR, MEMBRANOUS, CIRCULATORY, NERVOUS,

parturition aids REPRODUCTIVE, <u>NER-VOUS</u>, CIRCULATORY, MUSCULAR, GLANDULAR

pregnancy assistance <u>REPRODUCTIVE</u>, <u>CIRCU-LATORY</u>, <u>NERVOUS</u>, <u>GLAN-DULAR</u>, <u>DIGESTIVE</u>

prostate problems <u>URINARY</u>, <u>REPRODUC-TIVE</u>, <u>MUSCULAR</u>, GLAN-DULAR, CIRCULATORY, NERVOUS

sadism Perverted sexual pleasure of inflicting pain on others. <u>REPRODUCTIVE</u>, <u>GLAN-DULAR</u>, <u>NERVOUS</u>, DIGES-TIVE, URINARY/INTESTI-NAL

seminal/semen problems <u>REPRODUCTIVE</u>, <u>GLAN-DULAR</u>, CIRCULATORY, NERVOUS, DIGESTIVE

sex/sexual problems <u>REPRODUCTIVE</u>, <u>GLAN-DULAR</u>, CIRCULATORY, NERVOUS, DIGESTIVE, URINARY

spermatorrhea Abnormal involuntary loss of semen. <u>REPRODUCTIVE</u>, <u>NER-VOUS</u>, CIRCULATORY, GLANDULAR

spermoneuralgia

Pain in the testicles and spermatic cord.
<u>REPRODUCTIVE</u>, <u>NERVOUS</u>, CIRCULATORY, GLANDULAR

sterility

Inability to conceive offspring.
<u>REPRODUCTIVE</u>, <u>GLANDULAR</u>, <u>NERVOUS</u>, <u>CIRCULATORY</u>, <u>DIGESTIVE</u>

syphilis

Infectious veneral disease resulting in inflammation and ulcerations of skin and mucous membranes, and affecting other body organs and systems.
<u>GLANDULAR</u>, <u>MEMBRANOUS</u>/MUSCULAR, CIRCULATORY, REPRODUCTIVE, URINARY

testis/testicle problems

<u>REPRODUCTIVE</u>, <u>GLANDULAR</u>, CIRCULATORY, NERVOUS, MEMBRANOUS/ MUSCULAR, DIGESTIVE

uteritis

Inflammation of the uterus.
<u>MEMBRANOUS</u>, <u>GLANDULAR</u>, REPRODUCTIVE, CIRCULATORY

uterus/uterine problems

<u>REPRODUCTIVE</u>, <u>GLANDULAR</u>, NERVOUS, MEMBRANOUS, URINARY, DIGESTIVE

vaginal problems	REPRODUCTIVE, URINARY, MEMBRANOUS, GLANDULAR, CIRCULATORY, NERVOUS
vaginismus	Painful muscular contraction around the vagina. NERVOUS, REPRODUCTIVE, MUSCULAR, CIRCULATORY, GLANDULAR
vaginitis	Inflammation of the vagina or sheath. MEMBRANOUS, REPRODUCTIVE, CIRCULATORY, GLANDULAR
variocele	Enlargement of spermatic veins. REPRODUCTIVE, MEMBRANOUS, CIRCULATORY, GLANDULAR
venereal disease	Contagious social disease contracted generally by sexual intercourse. GLANDULAR, MEMBRANOUS, REPRODUCTIVE, CIRCULATORY, URINARY

CHAPTER SEVEN

HERBAL AID FOR ENERGIZING THE SUDORIFEROUS OR SWEAT GLANDS

Strengthened sweating function activates special cleansing/balancing of life fluids

The sudoriferous system (comprising sweat glands, excretory duct, sweat pores, and sweat centers in the nervous system) is responsible for stablizing the energy capabilities in your body's life fluids. These important body structures are involved with regulating body temperature (cooling via evaporation, warming via contraction of pores), elimination of body wastes (certain mineral salts, and proteinous/acid wastes), and aids blood nutrition into skin surfaces and an auxilliary intake of oxygen.

Balanced sudoriferous activity will efficiently regulate body heat and conserve the available energy resources. The sweat gland functions are needed to facilitate waste elimination, both blood and lymphatic overloads. Sweating deficiencies put serious stress upon the urinary and intestinal systems. Sudoriferous vitality is greatly aided by using selected aromatic herbs internally in the form of very warm teas and herb capsules taken with very warm water. Aromatic herbs will strongly activate sweating function by—

(1) influencing the sweat centers of the nervous system to function;

(2) activating circulation and drawing blood toward skin surfaces;

(3) enabling blood and lymphatic vessels to unburden impurities rapidly; and

(4) relieving stresses upon various eliminative channels—respiratory, urinary, intestinal.

Externally, these aromatic herbs are valued sudoriferous aids as fomentations, vapor baths, vapor packs, baths, washes, liniments, oils, footbaths, and the like (which are introduced in my HELP YOURSELF! textbook, Course 1). The herbal baths, vapor baths, and vapor packs are particularly valuable for aiding sudoriferous operations—relieving glands, energizing circulation, nourishing tissues, and strengthening respiration, and so forth.

Besides using selected herbal aids for the sudoriferous/sweat gland system, you will want to commit yourself to programs which will give balance to your lifestyle, including ample water, sunshine, and exercise. Unstable energies (hot or cold) signal a disruption of lifeline powers at some source. Sweating strengthens the processes of energy distribution, and energy resources are drawn into a problematic zone. Excessive heat, without sufficient moisture, is very disturbing to life line functions and is a destoyer of needed cells, while the combination of heat with ample fluids (internal and external) will have a salutary effect on general body capabilities and potentials! The sudoriferous/sweat gland system will enable your body's life line to attain optimum power with minimal encumberances, and it will restore the acid-alkaline balances for sustained physical performance!

Major characteristics of single herbs which supply sudoriferous aid

YARROW flowers, herb
Achillea millefolium

Powerful sweat gland activator; raises body heat and equalizes circulation; opens pores and relaxes the skin; activates glands and tones membranes

CAPSICUM or **CAYENNE** fruit
Capsicum annuum,
C. frutescens

One of nature's most powerful and persisting circulation activators (gives power to the pulse, equalizes blood flow in capillaries); strengthens tissues and activates secretions

ROSEMARY leaves
Rosmarinus officinalis

Reliable circulatory energizer and nervous balancer; skin/membranous activator

GINGER root
Zingiber officinale

Valuable activator of capillary circulation; nervous balancer; activates skin/membranous secretions

BAYBERRY rootbark
Myrica cerifera

Powerful circulation activator/cleanser (persisting influence on arteries and capillaries); strengthens skin/membrane secretions

Problems and malfunctions involving the sudoriferous/sweat gland system

communicable or contagious disease

SUDORIFEROUS/CIRCULATORY, GLANDULAR/URINARY/INTESTINAL, DIGESTIVE

epidemic diseases

Infectious disease or conditions reachng epidemic proportions in a geographical area. SUDORIFEROUS/CIRCULATORY, GLANDULAR, NERVOUS, URINARY/INTESTINAL

eruptive diseases

SUDORIFEROUS/CIRCULATORY, GLANDUALR, NERVOUS, URINARY/INTESTINAL, SKIN

fever

Abnormal rise of body temperature, usually accompanying other body disorders. CIRCULATORY/SUDORIFEROUS, GLANDULAR/

URINARY/INTESTINAL,
SKIN

hyperhidrosis

Excessive sweating.
NERVOUS, GLANDULAR,
CIRCULATORY

malaria, yellow fever

Parasitic invasion of red blood
cells resulting in periodic attacks of chills and fever, affecting digestive, nervous, and
glandular systems.
CIRCULATORY/SUDORI-
FEROUS, GLANDULAR,
NERVOUS, DIGESTIVE

measles, rubeola

Contagious catarrhal disorder,
resulting in distinct red circu-
lar eruption on the skin and
also mucous membranes of
the mouth (Koplik's spots), usually before adolescence.
CIRCULATORY/SUDORI-
FEROUS, GLANDULAR,
SKIN, NERVOUS

plague

Widespread epidemic disease
with high death rate.
SUDORIFEROUS/CIRCU-
LATORY, GLANDULAR,
NERVOUS, URINARY/IN-
TESTINAL

Q fever

Infectious disorder transmitted
by milk, contact with infected
animals, or ticks, resulting in
fever, chills, and muscular

pains.
SUDORIFEROUS/CIRCU-
LATORY, GLANDULAR,
NERVOUS, MUSCULAR,
DIGESTIVE

scarlet fever

Contagious febrile disorder,
resulting in mouth, nose, and
throat inflammation, a red rash,
and general toxemia.
SUDORIFEROUS/CIRCU-
LATORY, GLANDULAR,
MEMBRANOUS, URINARY/
INTESTINAL

smallpox, variola

Contagious, fever-producing
disorder, resulting in pustular
skin eruptions, sloughing and
scar formation.
SUDORIFEROUS/CIRCU-
LATORY, GLANDULAR,
SKIN, NERVOUS, URINARY/
INTESTINAL

spotted fever

Indicates various eruptive fe-
vers.
SUDORIFEROUS/CIRCU-
LATORY, GLANDULAR,
SKIN, NERVOUS, URI-
NARY/INTESTINAL

typhoid fever

Infectious fever-causing disease, resulting in lymphatic,
spleen and other glandular disturbances.
SUDORIFEROUS, GLAN-
DULAR, CIRCULATORY,
SKIN, NERVOUS, DIGES-

typhus fever

Infectious fever-causing disease resulting in nervous, circulatory, skin, intestinal, and urinary disorders.
SUDORIFEROUS/CIRCU-LATORY, GLANDULAR, SKIN, NERVOUS, URINARY/INTESTINAL, DIGESTIVE

varicella, chickenpox

Contagious disease resulting in a characteristic skin eruption.
SUDORIFEROUS/CIRCU-LATORY, GLANDULAR, SKIN, NERVOUS, URINARY/INTESTINAL

CHAPTER EIGHT

HERBAL AID FOR ENERGIZING THE DIGESTIVE SYSTEM (activating, soothing)

A healthy digestive appetite is the foundation to constitutional vigor

The digestive system (comprising various glandular secretions, stomach, and small intestines) is responsible for maintaining your body energies at a stable rate. A healthy appetite, which is an instinctive desire to replenish dynamic energies (organic life) depends on balanced body activity. A "nervous appetite" leads to malfunction; it originates with unresolved emotional stresses, induces excessive eating, and will result in overweight. A balanced program that includes dynamic energies from vigorous exercise will create a healthy appetite.

Loss of appetite relates to excess acidity in your body, and sodium foods (from various vegetables, greens, and herbs) are natural alkalinzers. Digestive vitality can become energized by using selected aromatic herbs internally in the form of warm teas and herb capsules taken with warm water. Aromatic herbs will enhance digestive funcitons by—

(1) activating circulatory functions to nourish vital digestive structures;

(2) sensitizing nervous responses within critical organs, glands, and tissues;

(3) promoting glandular secretions for catalyzing the essential digestive processes;

(4) balancing molecular reactions for arresting digestive fermentations and gas formation; and

(5) calming muscular malfunctions for relieving distress conditions.

Externally, these aromatic herbs are valuable digestive aids as fomentations, liniments, oils, vapors, baths, sitzbaths, and the like (which are introduced in my HELP YOURSELF! textbook, Course 1). Herbal liniments (external application of tinctures, extracts, and the like) and herbal sitzbaths are particularly useful for aiding nervous/muscular stress in the stomach. Aromatic herbs taken internally are invaluable for relieving general emotional stresses which greatly disturb local capillary circulation and production of digestive fluids within the stomach walls, and for balancing the muscular activities.

Besides using selected herbal aids for soothing activation of the digestive system, you will want to give your lifestyle adequate nervous/emotional balance and sufficient circulation and muscle tone by exercising, drinking ample water between meals, and eating wholesome (appetizing) foods. Your digestive system was intended to prepare increased life for your body and to make the whole health-building process delightfully appetizing and perpetually enjoyable!

Major characteristics of single herbs which supply digestive aid (activating, soothing)

GINGER root *Zingiber officinale*	Aids digestive secretions; soothes, counteracts putrefactions; acti-

vates circulation

CHAMOMILE flowers, herb
Matricaria chamomilla

One of the great digestive aids; also a restorer for circulatory nervous, respiratory, glandular, reproductive and muscular systems

WILD YAM root
Dioscorea villosa

Membranous cleanser, nervous balancer; counteracts putrefactions and removes obstructions; glandular and genitourinary aid

PAPAYA fruit, leaves
Carica papaya

Famous catalyst-restorer for digestive system (contains "papain"); also helpful for skin and muscular systems

PEPPERMINT herb
Mentha piperita

Digestive aid (counteracts fermentations and putrefactions); nerve calmative/tonic; general constitutional activator/restorer

SPEARMINT herb
Mentha viridis

Digestive aid; nerve calmative/ balancer; counteracts nauseous and vomiting tendencies; urinary activator/restorer

CATNIP herb
Nepeta cataria

Counteracts digestive/intestinal fermentations and putrefactions; nerve balancer/calmative, urinary activator

FENNEL seeds
Foeniculum vulgare

Reliable strengthening/soothing aid for digestion; balances nerves and glands (liver, spleen); covers bitter tastes; anti-cellulite aid for reducing

88

Basic herbal recipes (combinations) for supplying digestive aid (activating, soothing, calming, and so forth)

_____ papaya fruit, peppermint herb

_____ peppermint leaves, licorice root, cinnamon bark, spearmint leaves, (balm mint leaves)

_____ papaya fruit, ginger root, peppermint leaves, wild yam root, fennel seeds, lobelia herb, spearmint leaves, catnip herb, (clove flowers, coriander seed, myrrh gum)

_____ barberry rootbark, ginger root, cramp bark, fennel seeds, peppermint leaves, wild yam root, catnip herb, (wild ginger root, prickley ash bark, myrrh gum)

_____ gentian root, capsicum fruit, ginger root, wormwood herb, (clove flowers, wild yam root, myrrh gum)

Problems and malfunctions involving the digestive system (secretive activation, calming, and so on)

anorexia

Loss of appetite.
<u>DIGESTIVE</u>, NERVOUS, GLANDULAR

belching

Condition of gastric fermentation and escaping of gas from the stomach through the mouth.

colic

DIGESTIVE, NERVOUS, GLANDULAR

Spasmodic abdominal pain within a hollow or tubular soft organ.
DIGESTIVE, NERVOUS, GLANDULAR/INTESTINAL

flatulence, gas

Excessive gas in the stomach and intestines.
DIGESTIVE, NERVOUS, GLANDULAR

gastric problems

DIGESTIVE, MEMBRANOUS, NERVOUS, GLANDULAR

gastralgia

Stomach pain.
DIGESTIVE, NERVOUS, MEMBRANOUS, GLANDULAR

gastritis

Inflammation of the stomach.
MEMBRANOUS, DIGESTIVE, NERVOUS, GLANDULAR

heartburn

Burning discomfort behind the lower part of the sternum, resulting from excessive stomach acidity.
DIGESTIVE, GLANDULAR, MEMBRANOUS, NERVOUS, URINARY

indigestion, dyspepsia

Incomplete or imperfect digestion, resulting in upset stomach, acidity, gas, belching,

	and so on. DIGESTIVE, NERVOUS, GLANDULAR, URINARY
motion sickness	Nausea, dizziness, and vomiting induced by motion (especially travel by air, car, ship, and so forth). DIGESTIVE, NERVOUS, GLANDULAR
nausea	Stomach distress with a loathing for food and an urge to vomit. DIGESTIVE, NERVOUS, GLANDULAR

PART THREE

HERBAL AID FOR BUILDING/BALANCING/ REGENERATING BODY SYSTEMS
(using selected herbs with special bitter properties)

Bitter herbal aids are special resource foods for building general body constitution and balancing all metabolic activities:

DIGESTION is regenerated,
GLANDS (liver, lymphatics, spleen, and the like) are balanced, and
INTESTINES are restored.

Herbal aids to all these body systems have one characteristic in common: they are bitters that contain substances that are unpleasant to the taste. These constitutional and metabolic herbal aids are very powerful systemal restorers when taken in or with either cool or warm liquids. They are required for all difficult, distressing, and lingering malfunctions.

91

CHAPTER NINE

HERBAL AID FOR BUILDING/BALANCING THE DIGESTIVE OR GASTRO-INTESTINAL SYSTEM

Digestive vigor is the main source for body strength and vitality

The digestive tract (comprising stomach, small intestines, and related glands) is responsible for sustaining and maintaining body energies. If your resources of nutrition are adequate (meaning, that sufficient compounds are present in your foods and supplements for sustaining systemal energies, maintenance, and restoration), and if digestive structures and functions are reliable, then your whole body receives an increasing abundance of life power! When you fail to give proper care to your digestive system, you can expect trouble to develop somewhere. For sure, your stomach will either directly influence or indirectly be involved with the rise of most body malfunctions and ailments, even though it is usually the last to be suspected. All body systems depend on healthy digestion in order to replenish tissues, facilitate functions, repair structures, and promote metabolic balances.

Digestive harmony is strongly influenced by your own chosen lifestyle and nervous/emotional responses. Circulatory vigor and muscular tone are also vital to adequate glandular secretions and digestive activity. Your digestive capability can be strengthened by using bitter herbs internally in the form of (cool) herb teas and herb capsules taken with water. Bitter herbs will support and improve digestion by—

(1) enriching the glandular secretions so that digestive juices are effective;

(2) reinforcing the quality and quantity of enzymes which enable complete nutritional conversions;

(3) nourishing supportive tissues so that circulation, muscles, membranes, and the like, are active; and

(4) sustaining constitutional operations in all body parts so that your body has both endurance and resilience.

Externally, these bitter herbs (often in the form of aromatic bitters, such as wormwood herb, garden or wild sage herb, nettle leaves, rosemary leaves, and so on) are valuable digestive aids as fomentations, liniments, oils, baths, and sitzbaths (which are introduced in my HELP YOURSELF! textbook, Course 1). Herbal liniments and herbal sitzbaths with aromatic bitters are particularly useful for strengthening degenerating digestive conditions.

Besides using herbal aids internally and externally, you must also pay attention and take more care that your lifestyle is active and purposeful; make certain that you are achieving nervous/emotional balance; improve general circulation and local muscle tone through exercise; drink ample water between meals; eat wholesome (health-building) foods; and avoid ingesting harmful substances as much as possible. Also, do not forget to include some merry laughter at mealtimes, which is a great aid to digestion, circulation, and skin vitality. Your digestive system is designed to supply your body with an abundance of life. If this "fount" is clear and active, you can expect a steady supply of strength and vitality into all body systems and parts!

Major characteristics of single herbs which supply digestive aid

GENTIAN root
Gentiana lutea

Very effective and valued digestive aid; general constitutional restorer (high in organic oxygen); also useful for reproductive, glandular (liver, spleen), urinary, and muscular systems

ALFALFA herb
Medicago sativa

A valuable mineralizer and nutrient restorer for all body systems, with excellent absorptive capability

DANDELION root
Taraxacum officianle

Great blood-builder (high in potassium and other minerals); digestive restorer; valuable glandular builder (liver, spleen, pancreas); also urinary, reproductive, and skin restorer

GOLDEN SEAL root
Hydrastis canadensis

One of nature's most wonderful "cure-all" restorers (especially for crisis conditions); valuable antiseptic and decongestant for membranes; special strengthener of weakening muscular/skin tissues; valuable for digestive, glandular (liver), intestinal, respiratory, reproductive, and nervous malfunctions

MYRRH gum
Commiphora myrrha

One of the great constitutional restorers; useful for digestive, skin/membranous, intestinal, and other systems; antiseptic and invigorating for all stress and distress problems

IRISH MOSS plant
Chondrus crispus

One of nature's greatest constitutional mineralizers from the sea; general body alkalinizer, especially valued for glandular, digestive, skin/membranous, muscular/skeletal, and reproductive building and balancing

94

KELP plant
Macrosytic pyrifera

Great constitutional mineralizer from the sea, similar to Irish moss

WORMWOOD herb
Artemisia absinthium

Valued aromatic-bitter restorer; especially good stimulative tonic for all weak and feeble conditions; cleanses and firms tissues, removes obstructions

Basic herbal recipes (combinations) for supplying digestive aid

_____ comfrey root, pepsin, (myrrh gum) gentian root, capsicum fruit, ginger root, wormwood herb, (nettle leaves, agrimony root)

_____ kelp plant, dandelion root, alfalfa herb, (Irish moss plant, myrrh gum)

_____ golden seal root, capsicum fruit, myrrh gum, (eucalyptus leaves, clove flowers, wormwood herb)

_____ protein, capsicum fruit, rea clover tops, (myrrh gum, clove flowers)

_____ comfrey root, alfalfa herb, oatstraw, Irish moss plant, horsetail herb, lobelia herb, (clove flowers, red clover tops, dandelion root)

_____ kelp plant, Irish moss plant, parsley herb, capsicum fruit, (red clover tops, dandelion root, myrrh gum)

_____ comfrey leaves, wood betony herb, dandelion leaves, Siberian ginseng root, (papaya leaves)

_____ alfalfa herb, rose hips, chamomile flowers, psyllium seeds, dandelion root, bee pollen, myrrh gum, golden seal root, (papaya leaves, angelica root)

Problems and malfunctions involving the digestive system

abdominalgia

Abdominal pain.
DIGESTIVE, NERVOUS, MUSCULAR

alcoholism

Abnormal body conditions from excessive consumption of alcohol.
DIGESTIVE, GLANDULAR, NERVOUS, CIRCULATORY

96

caffeinism	Chronic effects from excessive use of coffee. DIGESTIVE, GLANDULAR, NERVOUS, CIRCULATORY
convalescence assistance	CIRCULATORY, DIGESTIVE, GLANDULAR, NERVOUS
deficiency disease	Disorder due to a lack of some essential nutritional substance. DIGESTIVE, GLANDUALR, CIRCULATORY
dietary assistance	DIGESTIVE, GLANDULAR, CIRCULATORY, NERVOUS, URINARY/INTESTINAL
digestion/digestive assistance	DIGESTIVE, GLANDULAR, CIRCULATORY, NERVOUS
dyspepsia, indigestion	Imperfect digestion, resulting in abdominal discomfort, loss of appetite and other irregularitites. CIRCULATORY, DIGESTIVE, GLANDULAR, NERVOUS
food poisoning	NEURO-EMETICS, CIRCULATORY/SUDORIFEROUS, GLANDULAR, DIGESTIVE, INTESTINAL

hunger, loss of	DIGESTIVE, CIRCULATORY, NERVOUS, GLANDULAR
kwashiorkor	Disorder resulting in protein malnutrition. DIGESTIVE, GLANDULAR
malnutrition	Faulty or inadequate nutrition, resulting from disorders of digestion, absorption, and distribution. DIGESTIVE, CIRCULATORY, GLANDULAR
mineral deficiencies	DIGESTIVE, GLANDULAR, CIRCULATORY, URINARY
nutrition/nutritive problems	DIGESTIVE, GLANDULAR, CIRCULATORY, NERVOUS
pellagra	Deficiency disorder associated with protein metabolism, resulting in gastro-intestinal, nervous, and other degenerations. DIGESTIVE, GLANDULAR, CIRCULATORY, MEMBRANOUS, SKIN, NERVOUS, URINARY/INTESTINAL
peptic ulcer	Ulcer in stomach wall irritated by digestive acids. MUSCULAR, DIGESTIVE, GLANDUALR, CIRULATORY, NERVOUS

98

poison/poisoning (antidote)	NERVOUS, GLANDULAR, MEMBRANOUS/MUSCULAR, DIGESTIVE
preventive maintenance	DIGESTIVE, CIRCULATORY, NERVOUS, GLANDULAR, MUSCULAR
putrefaction	Decomposition of tissue or animal matter, resulting in foul-smelling and poisonous products. DIGESTIVE, GLANDULAR, MUSCULAR, INTESTINAL
stomach problems	DIGESTIVE, MUSCULAR, CIRCULATORY, NERVOUS, GLANDULAR
vomiting or emesis	Ejection of stomach contents through the mouth. DIGESTIVE, NERVOUS, GLANDULAR, MEMBRANOUS

CHAPTER TEN

HERBAL AID FOR BUILDING/BALANCING THE GLANDULAR (EXOCRINE, ENDOCRINE) SYSTEM

Strong glandular operation will magnify your life-powers

The glandular system (comprising various secretive organs and cell-clusters—liver, lymphatic, adrenal, pancreas, spleen, gallbladder, gonads, thyroid, parathyroid, pituitary, pineal, thymus, and the like) is responsible for regulating and balancing body functions. These important glandular secretions influence, modify, and normalize all body activities and enable failing systems to become responsive and receptive to health-building resources. Healthy glands keep careful watch over all systemal operation, manufacture vital substances, store certain elements, regulate body functions, and detoxify the body's life line fluids (blood and lymph). Where glandular operations are properly balanced and effective, the blood-stream is clean, cells are healthy, and disease organisms have no place to propagate themselves. The glandular system is particularly needed to purify (filter) and discharge waste materials and foreign substances from the bloodstream and lymphatic channels. This important glandular function has been termed traditionally as "cleansing," "purifying," or "sweetening" the circulation.

Glandular harmony is very much interdependent on very delicate systemal interactions and balances. Glandular secretions are particularly sensitive and responsive to adequate mineralization (such as iodine, silicon, zinc, copper, iron, and so on). Your glandular capabilities can be strengthened by using bitter herbs in the form of (cool) herb teas and herb capsules taken with ample water. Bitter herbs will powerfully support and enhance glandular operations by—

(1) enriching the glandular secretions so that all body systems become sensitive and responsive to wholesome action;

(2) modifying the blood mineral composition so that it

100

maintains maximum life-carrying capability;

(3) restoring defective secretions so that body systems can regain harmony and balance, which will yield greater physical vibrancy;

(4) strengthening all metabolic potentials for more effective assimilation, metabolism, and elimination;

(5) giving powerful aid to the most difficult stress and lingering distress body conditions; and

(6) enabling hormone secretions to balance at optimum potency, which will reverse aging degenerations and restore body youthfulness.

Externally, the bitter herbs (often in the form of aromatic-bitters) are invaluable glandular aids as fomentations, liniments, oils, packs, baths, and vapor baths (which are introduced in my HELP YOURSELF! textbook, Course 1). Herbal oils, liniments, and vapor packs are particularly useful glandular aids, and you should not overlook the value of the herbal retention enema either.

Physical exercise is essential to healthy glandular functions. Dr. Bernard Jensen suggests that alternating tension/relaxation of the muscles (isometric exercises) around the various glands will aid both circulation and secretive functions. Remember, your glands are designed to oversee the unlimited computor-like complexities of your total body processes. Your glandular operations are very sensitive to your nervous/emotional states, and they function best when your lifestyle is balanced and purposive. Also, be aware that adequate exposure to air and water will invigorate the glands. Glandular balance will insure natural purity and continued vitality for all body systems, and your capabilities for life expression will be magnified beyond belief and understanding!

Major characteristics of single herbs which supply glandular aid

BURDOCK root *Arctium lappa*	One of nature's greatest blood cleansers and valued glandular restorers (liver, lymphatics);

special aid to skin/membranous and muscular tissues; also valuable for respiratory, urinary and intestinal systems

ECHINACEA or **PURPLE CONEFLOWER** root
Echinacea angustifolia

Powerful glandular restorer (liver, lymphatics); exceptional antiseptic and anti-infection herb; reliable aid for circulatory, digestive, skin, membranous, muscular, and reproductive systems

SARSAPARILLA root
Smilax medica and related species

Powerful glandular balancer and restorer, rich in organic minerals; reproductive strengthener (male and female hormones); also an effective aid for skin/membranous, muscular/skeletal, and urinary systems

LOBELIA herb, seeds
Lobelia inflata

One of the greatest glandular balancer/restorers in the herbal kingdom specifically recommended for stress and distress crisis conditions; especially valued for activating glands, nerves, membranes, and so on, and for removing problematic obstructions

BLACK WALNUT hulls, leaves
Juglans nigra

Great restorer for glandular (thyroid, liver, lymphatics), skin/membranous, muscular, reproductive, and intestinal systems; particularly helpful for persisting and distressing systemal malfunctions

CHAPARRAL herb
Larea tridentata,
L. mexicana

Famed Indian herb that is a powerful glandular cleanser/restorer (liver, lymphatics), especially for severe and degenerative problems; valued for skin/membranous and muscular/skeletal tissues, urinary and intestinal systems

GOLDEN SEAL root
Hydrastis canadensis

Considered to be a "cure-all" balancer/restorer for many disorders; valuable antiseptic and tissue builder (especially for weakness and congestion)

RED CLOVER blossoms
Trifolium pratense

Excellent glandular restorer, blood purifier and mineralizer (rich in calcium, silicon and trace elements); effective for severe skin/membranous, muscular, digestive, nervous, and respiratory malfunctions

LICORICE root
Glycyrrhiza glabra

Stimulates health-building glandular secretions (valuable hormone balancer); effective influence on all internal membranes and tissues (soothing, softening, lubricating, nourishing restorative)

YELLOW DOCK root
Rumex crispus

One of the great blood cleansing/building aids (high in organic iron); powerful glandular restorer (liver, lymphatics); also aids digestive, intestinal, skin/membranous, muscular, and respiratory systems

BARBERRY bark
Berberis vulgaris

Effective builder/restorer for glands (liver, spleen); also aids skin, respiratory, urinary, intestinal and other systems

DANDELION root
Taraxacum officinale

Valuable glandular builder/restorer (liver, spleen, pancreas), with special influence on digestion, urinary, skin, and other systems

PEACH bark
Amygdalus (Prunus) persica

Valued glandular activator and restorer to membranes and tissues; special aid to digestive, urinary, nervous, and respiratory systems

OREGON GRAPE root
Berberis aquifolium

Valuable blood purifier and liver activator; aids digestive, intestinal, genitourinary, and skin systems

STILLINGIA root
Stillingia sylvatica

Effective glanduluar activator (especially liver); aids skin, urinary, and respiratory systems

YUCCA root
Yucca glauca

Valued desert herb of Southwest Indians, with special influence on glandular (liver), skin, and muscular tissues, and respiratory and urinary systems

WATERCRESS herb
Nasturtium officinale

Valuable blood builder and glandular restorer (liver); also aids circulatory, urinary, and skin systems (rich in organic minerals)

VIOLET leaves
Viola odorata

A great glandular balancer/restorer; also useful for respiratory, nervous, digestive, and muscular systems

CHICKWEED herb
Stellaria media

Special restorer for blood vessels and hepatic veins for improved liver function; direct influence on all internal membranes and tissues

DESERT (BRIGHAM) TEA
Ephedra viridis and species

Valued restorer for glandular (high in organic copper), respiratory, muscular, circulatory, and genital systems

Basic herbal recipes (combinations) for supplying glandular aid

_____ gentian root, Irish moss plant, golden seal root, comfrey root, fenugreek seeds, safflower flowers, myrrh gum, yellow dock root, echinacea root, black walnut hulls, barberry root-bark, dandelion root, St. Johnswort herb, chickweed herb, catnip herb, cyani (cornflower) flowers, (blue flag root, burdock root, bladderwrack or seawrack plant, white ash bark, prickly ash bark, wild ginger root)

_____ chickweed herb, licorice root,

safflower flowers, echinacea root, black walnut hulls, gotu kola herb, hawthorn berries, papaya fruit, fennel seeds, dandelion root, (bladderwrack or seawrack plant, fenugreek seeds, blue flag root, burdock root, white ash bark, myrrh gum, prickly ash bark)

_____ licorice root, red clover tops, sarsaparilla root, cascara sagrada bark, Oregon grape root, chaparral herb, burdock root, buckthorn bark, prickly ash bark, peach bark, stillingia root, (blue flag root, wild ginger root, sanicle herb, spikenard root)

_____ protein, capsicum fruit, red clover tops, (prickly ash bark, myrrh gum, eucalyptus leaves, wild ginger root)

_____ yellow dock root, dandelion root, burdock root, licorice root, chaparral herb, red clover tops, barberry rootbark, cascara sagrada bark, yarrow herb, sarsaparilla root, (blue flag root, prickly ash bark, parsley root, golden seal root, spikenard root)

_____ echinacea root, golden seal root, yarrow flowers, capsicum fruit, (myrrh gum, clove flowers)

_____ echinacea root, yarrow leaves, myrrh gum, capsicum fruit, (eucalyptus leaves, thyme herb)

_____ red beet root, dandelion root, parsley herb, horsetail (shavegrass) herb, liverwort herb, birch leaves, lobelia herb, blessed thistle herb, angelica root, chamomile flowers, genetian root, goldenrod herb, (prickly ash bark, fringe tree bark, yellow dock root, burdock root)

_____ bromelain, yucca root, comfrey root, alfalfa herb, black cohosh root, yarrow flowers, capsicum fruit, chaparral herb lobelia herb, burdock root, centaury herb, (sanicle herb, boneset herb, parsley root, prickly ash bark, clove flower)

_____ hydrangea root, desert (Brigham) tea herb, chaparral herb, yucca root, black cohosh root, capsicum fruit, black walnut hulls, valerian root, sarsaparilla root, lobelia herb, scullcap herb, burdock root, wild lettuce leaves, wormwood herb, (wild ginger root, prickly ash bark, parsley root, boneset herb, bitter root root, blue flag root, clove flowers)

_____ kelp plant, Irish moss plant, parsley herb, capsicum fruit, (walnut hulls, nettle leaves, alfalfa leaves, blue flag root)

_____ Irish moss plant, kelp plant, black walnut hulls, parsley herb, watercress herb, sarsaparilla root, Iceland moss plant, (alfalfa leaves, nettle leaves, red clover tops, blue flag root)

_____ licorice root, safflower flowers, dandelion root, horseradish root, (nettle leaves, goldenrod herb, prickly ash bark, blue flag root, red clover tops)

_____ golden seal root, capsicum fruit, parsley root, desert (Brigham) tea herb, marshmallow root, chaparral herb, lobelia herb, burdock root, (echinacea root, eucalyptus leaves, chickweed herb, prickly ash bark)

Problems and malfunctions involving the glandular system

Addison's disease

Disease due to deficiency in adrenal cortical hormone secretions.
GLANDULAR, URINARY, CIRCULATORY, NERVOUS

adenalgia

Glandular pain.
GLANDULAR, NERVOUS, CIRCULATORY

adenitis

Inflammation of lymph nodes or gland.
GLANDULAR, <u>MEMBRAN-OUS</u>, CIRCULATORY

adiposis, cellulitis

Abnormal accumulation of body fat.
<u>GLANDULAR</u>, <u>URINARY</u>, CIRCULATORY, DIGESTIVE

adrenalitis, adrenitis

Inflammation of adrenal glands.
<u>GLANDULAR</u>, <u>URINARY</u>, CIRCULATORY

aging

Progressive body changes associated with growing old.
<u>GLANDULAR</u>, CIRCULATORY, NERVOUS, DIGESTIVE

allergy

Hypersensitivity and reaction of body tissues to a substance.
<u>GLANDULAR</u>, DIGESTIVE, NERVOUS

amaurosis

Loss of vision resulting from various abnormal body conditions.
<u>GLANDULAR</u>, <u>CIRCULATORY</u>, NERVOUS, URINARY/INTESTINAL

amblyopia

Reduced or dimmed vision due to other internal body conditions.
<u>GLANDULAR</u>, <u>CIRCULA-</u>

109

TORY, NERVOUS, URI-NARY/INTESTINAL

autointoxication
Condition caused by producing excessive body poisons.
GLANDULAR, URINARY, INTESTINAL, DIGESTIVE

biliousness
Disordered liver condition resulting in constipation, headache, loss of appetite and vomiting of bile.
GLANDULAR, CIRCULATORY, DIGESTIVE

cachexia
Wasting condition of ill health associated with tuberculosis, cancer, and glandular irregularities.
GLANDULAR, DIGESTIVE, CIRCULATORY, MEMBRANOUS/MUSCULAR

cell metabolism problems
GLANDULAR, CIRCULATORY, NERVOUS, MUSCULAR, DIGESTIVE

cholera
Infectious disease with severe diarrhea, cramps, and loss of body fluids.
GLANDULAR, MEMBRANOUS, NERVOUS, CIRCULATORY, DIGESTIVE

cirrhosis
Chronic liver disorder with excessive connective tissue formation, contraction and hardening, resulting in tissue de-

generation, decrease in function, and increased resistance to blood flow through the liver.
GLANDULAR, CIRCULATORY, MUSCULAR, NERVOUS, DIGESTIVE

crisis condition

Critical period of body resources and energies, often signaling the maximum point of impurity expulsions after which body systems can begin to gain strength and normalize.
CIRCULATORY/SUDORIFEROUS, NERVOUS, GLANDULAR, URINARY/INTESTINAL, DIGESTIVE

Cushing's disease

Obesity, muscular weakness, and other disorders associated with excessive adrenal secretions and over-stimulation of the pituitary gland.
GLANDULAR, URINARY, CIRCULATORY, DIGESTIVE

cystic fibrosis

Glandular derangements of infants to young adults affecting all glands, particularly pancreas and sweat glands.
GLANDULAR, CIRCULATORY, DIGESTIVE

degeneration problems

CIRCULATORY, NERVOUS, MUSCULAR/SKELETAL, DIGESTIVE, GLANDULAR, URINARY/INTESTINAL

diabetes mellitus	Pancreatic disorder of carbo-hydrate metabolism and insufficient insulin production. GLANDULAR, DIGESTIVE, CIRCULATORY, URINARY
distress	Physical or mental suffering, condition of intense trouble and desperate need for aid. GLANDULAR, CIRCULATORY, NERVOUS, DIGESTIVE, URINARY/INTESTINAL
drug withdrawal	GLANDULAR, NERVOUS, CIRCULATORY, DIGESTIVE, URINARY/INTESTINAL
ear problems	GLANDULAR, CIRCULATORY, NERVOUS, URINARY
emotion/emotional problems	GLANDULAR, NERVOUS, CIRCULATORY, DIGESTIVE
endocrine problems	GLANDULAR, CIRCULATORY, NERVOUS, DIGESTIVE
endurance problems	GLANDULAR, CIRCULATORY, NERVOUS, DIGESTIVE
enzyme problems	DIGESTIVE, GLANDULAR, CIRCULATORY
fat problems	Adipose, obese, or corpulent condition. GLANDULAR, CIRCULA-

TORY, URINARY, DIGES-
TIVE, MUSCULAR

gallbladder problems

GLANDULAR, CIRCULA-
TORY, MEMBRANOUS,
NERVOUS

gallstone

Concretion or stone formed in
the gallbladder or bile ducts.
GLANDULAR, MEMBRAN-
OUS, CIRCULATORY, NER-
VOUS

gland problems

GLANDULAR, CIRCULA-
TORY, NERVOUS, DIGES-
TIVE

goiter

Enlargement of the thyroid
gland due to inflammation,
infection, or tumor.
GLANDULAR, MUSCULAR,
CIRCULATORY, NERVOUS,
DIGESTIVE

hepatic, liver problems

GLANDULAR, CIRCULA-
TORY, NERVOUS, MUSCU-
LAR, DIGESTIVE

hepatitis

Inflammation of the liver.
GLANDULAR, MEMBRAN-
NOUS, CIRCULATORY,
NERVOUS, DIGESTIVE,
URINARY

Hodgkin's disease

Enlargement of lymphatic tissue, spleen, and liver, with
lymphoid invasion into other
tissues.

113

GLANDULAR, CIRCULA-TORY, URINARY, DIGES-TIVE

hormone imbalance

GLANDULAR, REPRO-DUCTIVE, DIGESTIVE

hypoglycemia

Glandular disorder resulting in blood sugar deficiency, accompanied by functional weakness and irritability.
GLANDULAR, CIRCULA-TORY, NERVOUS, DIGES-TIVE

jaundice, icterus

Excess bile in the blood resulting in yellowish skin pigmentation, from liver and bile duct disorders.
GLANDULAR, CIRCULA-TORY, URINARY

liver problems

GLANDULAR, CIRCULA-TORY, MUSCULAR, NER-VOUS, DIGESTIVE

longevity potenitial

Capacity for continuing long life.
GLANDULAR, DIGESTIVE, CIRCULATORY, NERVOUS

lymphatic problems

GLANDULAR, MEMBRAN-OUS, CIRCULATORY, DI-GESTIVE, INTESTINAL

malignancy

Cancerous tumor.
GLANDULAR, MUSCULAR,

Malta fever, undulant fever Infectious disease transmitted from animals, affecting the spleen, lymphatic joints, with weakness and reoccurring attacks of fever.
GLANDULAR, CIRCULATORY/SUDORIFEROUS, NERVOUS, DIGESTIVE

metabolism problems GLANDULAR, CIRCULATORY, NERVOUS, DIGESTIVE

mumps Contagious viral disorder, resulting in inflammation of parotid and other salivary glands.
GLANDULAR, MUSCULAR, CIRCULATORY

pancreas/pancreatic problems GLANDULAR, DIGESTIVE, CIRCULATORY, NERVOUS, MUSCULAR

pancreatitis Pancreas inflammation and functional disorder
GLANDULAR, MUSCULAR, CIRCULATORY, NERVOUS

pernicious anemia Severe blood disorder resulting in a decrease in number and an increase in the size of red blood cells, accompanied by digestive deficiency, muscular weakness, nervous and skin irregularities, and so forth.

GLANDULAR, DIGESTIVE,
MUSCULAR, CIRCULA-
TORY, NERVOUS

pituitary problems

GLANDULAR, NERVOUS,
CIRCULATORY, DIGES-
TIVE

ptyalism

Excessive salivary secretions.
GLANDULAR, MEMBRAN-
OUS, DIGESTIVE, NERVOUS

puerperal fever

Blood poisoning resulting from
local uterine infection following
childbirth, accompanied with
chills, fever, and general prostration.
GLANDULAR, MUSCULAR,
CIRCULATORY, NERVOUS,
REPRODUCTIVE

pyemia

Infectious blood poisoning, re-
sulting in multiple spreading
abscesses in various body parts.
GLANDULAR, MUSCULAR,
CIRCULATORY, DIGES-
TIVE, URINARY

salivary problems

GLANDULAR, MEMBRAN-
OUS, NERVOUS, CIRCULA-
TORY, DIGESTIVE

scrofula

Infectious swelling of lympha-
tic glands in the neck, tubercu-
losis of lymphatic glands.
GLANDULAR, CIRCULA-
TORY, MEMBRANOUS,
URINARY

septicemia, sepsis	Blood poisoning from a source of infection, resulting in chills, fever and prostration. GLANDULAR, SUDO-RIFEROUS/CIRCULATORY, MUSCULAR, URINARY
spleen problems	GLANDULAR, CIRCULA-TORY, MUSCULAR, DIGES-TIVE, NERVOUS, URINARY
splenitis	Spleen inflammation, enlarge-ment, pain. GLANDULAR, MUSCULAR, CIRCULATORY, NERVOUS, URINARY
thymus problems	GLANDULAR, CIRCULA-TORY, NERVOUS
thyroid problems	GLANDULAR, CIRCULA-TORY, NERVOUS
toxemia	Abnormal presence of poi-sionous bacterial products in the blood. GLANDULAR, URINARY/ INTESTINAL, CIRCULA-TORY, DIGESTIVE

117

CHAPTER ELEVEN

HERBAL AID FOR BUILDING/BALANCING THE INTESTINAL (particularly lower bowel) SYSTEM

Efficient intestinal action helps your body retain its energy charge

The intestinal system (including the small intestines, but particularly the large intestines comprising the cecum and appendix, colon, and rectum) is responsible for removing resistance substances (such as metabolic wastes and toxins) from your body's lifeline channels. Your body's energy resources are greatly enhanced by its purity and by an efficient removal of metabolic residues. There is a direct relationship between the rate of intestinal decomposition/elimination and the degree of health achieved elsewhere in your body. A sluggish colon will give rise to stagnation, putrefaction, and reabsorption of highly toxic materials which precipitate numerous local problems and various general body malfunctions. Dr. Bernard Jensen in one of his books quotes the noted British physician, Sir Arbuthnot Lane, to the effect that the lower intestinal tract should be emptied via bowel movement at least every six hours in order to maintain eliminative efficiency and to avoid impurity build-up and aging degenerations within your body.

Intestinal vitality is sustained by a varied and balanced diet, which includes sufficient fiber and cleansing compounds that are present in fresh vegetables, leafy greens, fruits, and selected herbs. The intestines are really an extension of your digestive system, and *intestinal weakness usually begins in the stomach* (particularly from an insufficiency of hydrochloric secretions, accompanied by liver and bile imbalances). Good intestinal function requires adequate circulation, nervous power, and tissue tone. Your intestinal capability can be strengthened by using bitter herbs internally in the form of (cool) herb teas and herb capsules taken with ample water. Bitter herbs will powerfully support and activate intestinal operations by—

(1) strengthening glandular secretions so that metabolic

wastes are processed and discharged efficiently;

(2) stabilizing intestinal juices to improve the retension and growth of favorable or "friendly" bacteria;

(3) nourishing structures so that intestinal action is vigorous and sustained;

(4) supplying adequate organic compounds which help arrest detrimental fermentations and putrefactions;

(5) counteracting alkalinizing conditions which are conducive to parasitic infestation; and

(6) cleansing parasitic conditions.

Externally, the bitter herbs (often in the form of aromatic bitters) are invaluable intestinal aids as fomentations, liniments, oils, baths, vapor baths, sitzbaths, and the like, (which are introduced in the HELP YOURSELF! textbook, Course 1). Sitzbaths, rectal injections, and cleansing enemas are particularly useful intestinal aids.

Two factors are very important for helping you to establish good intestinal function: exercise and rest. Your body's functions are cyclic, and it does its most effective cleansing during periods of rest. When your body does not receive the best grade of food and this low grade input is not metabolized efficiently, there will be a greater burden and stress put upon eliminative channels. Also, the rest factor will become even more important. Exercise is vital for circulatory vigor, glandular activity, and muscular tone; these are essential for elimination efficiency in the intestinal tract. A body that does not get a cyclic systemal cleansing and a recharge of its regular energy potentials will slowly run down and open itself to an increasing number of problems and malfunctions!

Major characteristics of single herbs which supply intestinal aid

CASCARA SAGRADA or **SACRED BARK** bark *Rhamnus purshiana*	One of nature's best intestinal restorers; also excellent for digestive, glandular (liver, pancreas, and so on), and nervous systems

119

RHUBARB root
*Rheum palmatum,
R. officianale, R.
rhaponticum*

Great restorer for the intestines (especially suited for children as well as adults); also valued for glandular (liver, gall ducts), digestive, and membranous systems

BUCKTHORN bark
Rhamnus frangula

Valuable restorer for the intestines (including antiparasitic cleanser); valued also for glandular (liver), urinary, skin, and muscular systems

ALOE leaves (resin)
*Aloe vera, A. perryi,
A. ferox,* and species

Excellent intestinal restorer; also reliable for glandular (liver, spleen), digestive, urinary, genital, skin/membranous, and muscular systems

PSYLLIUM seeds
Plantago psyllium

Very valuable intestinal cleanser/balancer/restorer (soothes and relieves internal stresses of toxicity); special aid to digestion and membranes

CULVER'S ROOT or
TALL SPEEDWELL root
*Veronica virginica,
Leptandra virginica*

Powerful intestinal aid and restorer; valuable for glandular (liver), digestive, and skin/membranous systems

LICORICE root
Glycyrrhiza glabra

Effective restorer for internal membranes and tissues (increases secretions, lubricates and nourishes the intestinal tract); valuable as a glandular aid (hormone balancer) and respiratory strengthener; modifies action and covers the taste of other bitters

Basic herbal recipes (combinations) for supplying intestinal aids

_____ cascara sagrada bark, buckthorn bark, licorice root, capsicum fruit, ginger root, barberry rootbark, couchgrass herb, red clover tops, lobelia herb, (black walnut leaves, butternut bark, marshmallow root)

_____ cascara sagrada bark, rhubarb root, golden seal root, capsicum fruit, ginger root, barberry rootbark, lobelia herb, fennel seeds, red raspberry, (psyllium seeds, bitter root, myrrh gum)

_____ pumpkin seeds, Culver's root, violet leaves, comfrey root, cascara sagrada bark, witch hazel bark, mullein leaves, slippery elm bark, (wormwood herb, pomegranate rootbark, male fern root, tansy herb, butternut bark)

121

Problems and malfunctions involving the intestinal system

amebiasis

Parasitic infection due to amoeba.
<u>INTESTINAL</u>, <u>MEMBRAN-OUS</u>, <u>GLANDULAR</u>

appendicitis

Inflammation of the appendix.
<u>MEMBRANOUS</u>, <u>GLANDU-LAR</u>, <u>NERVOUS</u>

autotoxemia, autotoxicosis

Self-poisoning due to absorption of body toxins.
<u>INTESTINAL</u>, <u>GLANDU-LAR</u>, <u>URINARY</u>, <u>CIRCULA-TORY</u>

bowel problems

<u>INTESTINAL</u>, <u>GLANDULAR</u>, DIGESTIVE, CIRCULA-TORY, MEMBRANOUS

celiac disease

Condition of intestinal malabsorption.
<u>MEMBRANOUS</u>, <u>GLANDU-LAR</u>, <u>INTESTINAL</u>, CIRCU-LATORY, DIGESTIVE

colitis, colonitis

Inflammation of colon, and can develop into mucous membrane disorder and degeneration.
<u>MEMBRANOUS</u>, <u>GLANDU-LAR</u>, DIGESTIVE, INTES-TINAL, CIRCULATORY

colon problems	MEMBRANOUS, GLANDULAR, INTESTINAL, DIGESTIVE, CIRCULATORY
constipation, costiveness	Difficult, delayed, and infrequent passage of hard and dry fecal material. INTESTINAL, CIRCULATORY, MEMBRANOUS (mucilages), DIGESTIVE/ GLANDULAR
defecation problems	INTESTINAL, CIRCULATORY, MEMBRANOUS, GLANDULAR
diarrhea	Gastro-intestinal disturbance resulting in frequent and watery bowel movements. MEMBRANOUS (astringents), DIGESTIVE/GLANDULAR, CIRCULATORY
diverticulitis	Inflammation of intestinal diverticula, particularly in the colon causing fecal stagnations in the destended sacs. MEMBRANOUS (mucilages), GLANDULAR, CIRCULATORY, DIGESTIVE/INTESTINAL
duodenal/duodenum problems	CIRCULATORY, MEMBRANOUS, DIGESTIVE, GLANDULAR

dysentery

Infectious intestinal disorder with severe inflammation of mucous membrane, diarrhea, and passage of mucous and blood.
MEMBRANOUS, CIRCULATORY, DIGESTIVE/GLANDULAR

elimination problems

INTESTINAL/DIGESTIVE/ GLANDULAR, CIRCULATORY

enteritis

Intestinal inflammation, affecting mucous and sub-mucous tissues.
MEMBRANOUS, CIRCULATORY, GLANDULAR, DIGESTIVE

evacuation/excretion problems

INTESTINAL/GLANDULAR, DIGESTIVE, CIRCULATORY, MEMBRANOUS (mucilages)

hemorrhoid(s), piles

Mass of dilated and painful veins in swollen tissue near the anus.
MUSCULAR, GLANDULAR/ INTESTINAL, CIRCULATORY, NERVOUS, DIGESTIVE

intestinal problems	INTESTINAL/GLANDULAR/ DIGESTIVE, MEMBRANOUS, CIRCULATORY
parasites	Unwanted, debilitating organisms living at the expense of body functions. GLANDULAR/INTESTNAL, DIGESTIVE, CIRCULATORY, NERVOUS, URINARY
proctitis, rectitis	Inflammation of the rectum and anus. MEMBRANOUS, GLANDULAR/INTESTINAL, CIRCULATORY, NERVOUS
rectal/rectum problems	MEMBRANOUS, CIRCULATORY, GLANDULAR/INTESTINAL, NERVOUS, DIGESTIVE
tapeworm, taenia	INTESTINAL/GLANDULAR, DIGESTIVE
worm problems	INTESTINAL/GLANDULAR, DIGESTIVE

PART FOUR
HERBAL AID FOR CLEANSING AND BEAUTI-FYING/SUPPORTING BODY SYSTEMS (using selected herbs with special cosmetic/cleansing, astringent or mucilaginous properties)

Cosmetic/cleansing herbal aids are special resource foods for removing unwanted waste accumulations from internal and external surfaces. These herbs are the "tissue toners" that give your body its radiance, posture, and expressive beauty:

SKIN and MEMBRANES are refreshed, and
MUSCLES and SKELETON are strengthened.

Herbal aids to the beautifying/supportive body systems are tissue cleansers and cosmetics, which have at least one of two characteristics in common: they contain astringing organic acids (astringents), or they contain slimy mucilages and fixed oil (demulcents). These herbal aids are effective taken with either cool or warm liquids. They should be greatly emphasized when your body is in a state of crisis from excess impurities or toxins and when a special cleansing procedure is needed.

CHAPTER TWELVE

HERBAL AID FOR CLEANING/BEAUTIFYING THE SKIN AND MEMBRANOUS SYSTEMS

Clean membranes and vibrant skin are natural expressions of your total beauty care

The skin and membranous coverings constitute the largest organ of your body. These important systems, while easily recognized as protective and beautifying surfaces, are often overlooked for their value to internal health building. Some of the vital skin/membranous functions are external beautificaton, internal cleanliness, surface protection, heat regulation, sense stimulation, nervous sensitivity, moisture balance, and tissue oxygenation. There is a very close relationship between skin/membranous vitality that is indicative of the presence of (or lack of) vibrancy within internal structures, functions, and balances. A balanced skin/membranous temperature over the entire body is a sign of good circulation, and this salutary condition requires enriched healthy blood and lymph that is energized, purified, oxygenized, and mineralized. Skin/membranous temperature is your "natural body thermostat"—when your temperature becomes excessively high (such as general fever or local congestion), it is a sign of impurities and foreign substances invading the body; when your temperature becomes excessively low (such as general chill or cold extemities and parts), it is a sign of circulatory or neuro/muscular weakness. Your natural skin/membranous temperature will feel "comfortably cozy and warm" when your body is filled with a balanced flow of nutrient energies to all parts.

Again, skin/membranous degenerations and unpleasant odors relate to unwholesome internal conditions and imbalances. Healthy external skin and internal membranes serve as important alkaline-acid balancers to your body, and will actively relieve impurity stresses within other systems and parts. Skin/membrane tissues can be cleansed and beautified by using cosmetic herbs internally in the form of (cool) teas and herb capsules taken with ample water, along with your externally applied herbal skin products. Cosmetic herbs will support skin/membranous operation by—

(1) removing negative impurities from tissue surfaces so that body polarities are balanced and energies are dynamic;

(2) strengthening cellular structures so that surfaces are elastic and resilient;

(3) balancing warmth, mositure, lubrication, and secretions of tissues;

(4) supplying needed mineralization and oxygenation so that cellular functions remain active and youthful; and

(5) arresting degenerations, catalyzing restorations, and promoting rejuvenation within all body systems. Externally, these cosmetic/cleansing herbs are valuable skin/membranous aids as creams, lotions, packs, oils, liniments, poultices, vapors, baths, and washes (which are introduced in my **HELP YOURSELF**! texbook, Course 1). Herbal beauty care is not merely skin deep! Skin/membrane vibrancy is the result of healthful body energies overflowing with life-nutrients into exterior surfaces! The various malfunctions that result in aging, drying, wrinkling, and so forth have their real origins in digestive, glandular (expecially liver and lymphatic), circulatory, urinary/intestinal, and other systemal disorders.

Besides using selected herbal aids for supplying "nature's natural look" to skin/membranous surfaces, you must remember that beautiful skin and healthy membranes are the result of treating your body well. You cannot abuse the surfaces or the interior of your physical temple without marring the beauty and responsiveness of its countenance! Exercise is essential, along with adequate nutrition and rest, regular exposure to air, sunshine, and water, skin brushing, massage therapy, clay packs, and the like, for achieving optimum skin/membranous radiance and attractiveness. Your skin and membranes were meant to mirror the expressive beauty created within your body and soul, and you skin was especially designed to achieve maximum artistry for pleasant social interactions!

Major characteristics of single herbs which supply skin/membranous aid

ALOE VERA gel (resin)
Aloe vera

Valuable cleanser/restorer for distressed tissues (specific for burns)

COMFREY root
Symphytum officinale

One of nature's greatest tissue builders; contains allatoin which promotes rapid cell production

GOLDEN SEAL root
Hydrastis canadensis

One of nature's most wonderful tissue restorers (valuable antiseptic), with special influence on congested membranes and weakening tissues

MYRRH gum
Commiphora myrrha

Important activator of circulatory capillaries; tissue activator and strengthener (excellent antiseptic and disinfectant)

BAYBERRY rootbark
Myrica cerifera

Powerful stimulating/cleansing/strengthening aid; one of nature's best herbs for obstructive conditions (contains valuable organic acids, gums, and resins for cleansing and restorative purposes)

CHICKWEED herb
Stellaria media

Excellent soothing/cleansing/strengthening aid to disordered and distressed skin and membranes.

WHITE OAK bark
Quercus alba
and related species

Powerful tissue cleanser/strengthener, antiseptic and disinfectant; counteracts poisons and venoms

WITCH HAZEL leaves, bark
Hamamelis virginiana

Valued for cleansing and strengthening tissue; useful aid for highly disordered surfaces

EYEBRIGHT herb
Euphrasia officinale

Reliable cleanser/restorer to delicate membranes and tissues

FENUGREEK seeds
Trigonella foenum-graecum

Excellent tissue restorer; functional aid to skin/membranous and muscular systems

OAT straw
Avena sativa

Important skin and membrane aid; rich in organic silicon

Basic herbal recipes (combinations) for supplying skin and membranous aid

_____ comfrey root, fenugreek seeds, (chickweed herb, elecampane root)

_____ golden seal root, bayberry rootbark, eyebright herb, (corn flowers, marigold flowers)

_____ bayberry rootbark, ginger root, white pine bark, capsicum fruit, clove flowers, (hemlock spruce tree bark, prickly ash bark, myrrh gum)

_____ golden seal root, capsicum fruit, myrrh gum, (eucalyptus

130

leaves, clove flowers)

_____   comfrey root, golden seal root, slippery elm bark, aloe leaves (resin), (ground ivy leaves, myrrh gum)

_____   golden seal root, bayberry root-bark, eyebright herb, red raspberry leaves, capsicum fruit, (chickweed herb, myrrh gum)

Problems and malfunctions involving the skin and membranous systems

abrasion

Injury by scraping away of a portion of skin or mucous membrane.
SKIN/MEMBRANOUS, NERVOUS, CIRCULATORY

acne

Inflammatory disease of oil glands and hair follicles of skin, marked by papules and pustules on the face (especially adolescents).
SKIN, GLANDULAR

Albert's disease, osteitis fibraosa cystica

Pigmentations and tumorous condition of skin.
GLANDULAR, SKIN

alopecia, acomia

Partial or complete hair deficiency baldness.
SKIN, GLANDULAR, CIRCULATORY

anaphia

Altered (diminished, loss of)

sense of touch.
NERVOUS, SKIN, GLAN-
DULAR

angiokeratoma
Skin disorder of feet and legs, with warty growths and thickening of skin along dilated capillaries.
SKIN, GLANDULAR, CIRCULATORY

aptha, thrush
Small ulcer on a mucous membrane in the mouth.
MEMBRANOUS, GLANDULAR

athlete's foot
Fungus infection and inflammation of skin around the toes and ball of the foot.
SKIN, GLANDULAR

baldness
(see alopecia)

bedsore
Local ulceration over a bony prominence usually due to lengthy confinement in bed.
SKIN, CIRCULATION

bite or sting
Injury by insects or animals in which body surfaces are torn, often becoming infected and may contain venoms.
SKIN (local astringent), GLANDULAR, NERVOUS

blister
A collection of fluid or serum below the skin from a pressure or a burn.

132

body odor

Displeasing body scent arising from digestive disorders, excessive body wastes and toxins in circulation, sweat secretions, and so forth.
DIGESTIVE/GLANDULAR, URINARY/INTESTINAL, SKIN, CIRULATORY

callus

Abnormal thickening of a skin layer.
SKIN, GLANDULAR, CIRCULATORY

canker, aptha

Painful white spots on mucous membrane of the mouth.
MEMBRANOUS, GLANDULAR, CIRCULATORY

cataract

Clouding of the lens and/or its capsule, obstructing the passage of light.
MEMBRANOUS, GLANDULAR, CIRCULATORY

cellulitis

Inflammation of cellular or connective tissue.
MEMBRANOUS, CIRCULATORY, URINARY/GLANDULAR

chafing

Slight inflammation of the skin due to friction from clothing or adjacent skin.
SKIN

chickenpox, varicella

Mild, contagious disease manifesting eruptions on skin and mucous membranes.
<u>SUDORIFEROUS</u>, <u>GLAN-DULAR</u>, MEMBRANOUS/SKIN, NERVOUS

cleansing (to facilitate)

CIRCULATORY/<u>SUDORI-FEROUS</u>, <u>URINARY</u>/<u>GLANDULAR</u>/<u>INTESTINAL</u>

conjunctivitis

Inflammation of mucous membrane lining the eyelids.
<u>MEMBRANOUS</u>, <u>CIRCULA-TORY</u>, <u>GLANDULAR</u>
(local and internal)

cosmetic aids

<u>CIRCULATORY</u>, <u>SKIN</u>, <u>GLANDULAR</u>

cut(s)

Penetration of skin or muscular tissue with a sharp-edged instrument.
<u>SKIN</u>/<u>MUSCULAR</u>, CIRCU-LATORY, NERVOUS

cyanosis

Skin discoloration (bluish, grayish, purplish) by reduced hemoglobin in the blood, resulting in poor oxygenation of the tissues.

dandruff, scurf

Abnormal peeling or scaling of skin on the scalp, sometimes due to irregularities of the sebaceous glands.
<u>GLANDULAR</u>, <u>CIRCULA-TORY</u>, SKIN

deodorant assistance
SKIN (local astringent), GLANDULAR/URINARY/INTESTINAL, CIRCULATORY

dermatitis
Inflammation of the skin, with redness, irritation, itching, and possible eruptions.
SKIN, GLANDULAR, CIRCULATORY

eczema
Chronic dermatitis or inflammatory skin condition with redness, itching, oozing eruptions, scaling, crusting, scabbing, and so forth.
SKIN, GLANDULAR, CIRCULATORY, URINARY/INTESTINAL

elephantiasis
Excessive growth and thickening of skin and sub-skin tissues from obstructed lymphatic vessels.
GLANDULAR, SKIN/MUSCULAR, CIRCULATORY

epidermis, skin problems
SKIN, GLANDULAR, CIRCULATORY, URINARY/INTESTINAL

erysipelas
Systemic feverish disturbance manifesting localized skin redness from inflammation and swelling.
GLANDULAR, CIRCULATORY, SKIN, URINARY/INTESTINAL

erythema

Spotty redness difused over the skin from capillary congestion. CIRCULATORY, GLANDULAR, SKIN

eye problems

MEMBRANOUS, CIRCULATORY, GLANDULAR, NERVOUS

face problems

SKIN, CIRCULATORY, GLANDULAR, NERVOUS

frostbite

Freezing or cold nipping of a body part, such as fingers, toes, nose causing tingling, redness, numbness, and circulation/tissue degeneration. CIRCULATORY, SKIN/MUSCULAR, NERVOUS, GLANDULAR

hair problems

SKIN, GLANDULAR, CIRCULATORY

Hansen's disease

(see leprosy)

herpes, cold sore, fever blister

Infectious disorder marked by blister formations on the skin or mucous membrane. MEMBRANOUS/SKIN (astringent), GLANDULAR

hives, urticaria

Allergic reaction, causing itchy areas of swelling on the skin or mucous membranes. GLANDULAR/DIGESTIVE, NERVOUS

impetigo

Contagious inflammatory skin disorder, with isolated pustules with yellowish crusts, principally around the mouth and nostrils.
SKIN, GLANDULAR

insect bites and stings

Venom and toxic response from bite or sting.
SKIN (astringent), GLANDULAR, NERVOUS

itching, pruritis

Skin irritation.
SKIN, NERVOUS, GLANDULAR, URINARY/INTESTINAL

lupus

Chronic progressive skin disorders with lesions or ulcers.
SKIN, GLANDULAR, CIRCULATORY

membrane problems

MEMBRANOUS, CIRCULATORY, DIGESTIVE, GLANDULAR

mole

Small permanent, discolored spot that is elevated above the surface of the skin.
GLANDULAR, SKIN, CIRCULATORY

mucus

Viscous fluid secretion of the mucous membranes, excessive secretions and congestions associated with circulatory impurities, membranous disorders, and so on.

137

	MEMBRANOUS, CIRCU-LATORY, GLANDULAR, URINARY/INTESTINAL
nose problems	MEMBRANOUS/MUSCU-LAR, GLANDULAR, CIR-CULATORY
odor	(see body odor)
peritonitis	Inflammation of the perito-neum or the serious membrane lining the abdominal cavity. MEMBRANOUS, GLANDU-LAR, CIRCULATORY, URINARY
perspiration problems	SKIN/SUDORIFEROUS, GLANDULAR, CIRCULA-TORY, NERVOUS, DIGES-TIVE
pityriasis	Sever skin disorder with dry branny scales or scurfy red patches. SKIN, GLANDULAR, CIR-CULATORY
poison ivy, oak, sumac	SKIN (astringents), GLAN-DULAR, CIRCULATORY, NERVOUS
polyp(s)	Projecting mass of swollen or tumorous membrane in the nose, uterus, or rectum. MEMBRANOUS (astringents), GLANDULAR, CIRCULA-TORY

prickly heat	Eruption of red pimples around sweat ducts, especially during hot weather, resulting in intense itching and tingling of affected parts. SKIN, GLANDULAR, CIRCULATORY, NERVOUS
proud flesh	Excessive growth of granulation when tissue does not heal or scab. SKIN/MUSCULAR, GLANDULAR, CIRCULATORY
prurigo	Persisting inflammatory skin disorder, resulting in recurring intensely-itching papules. SKIN, GLANDULAR, CIRCULATORY, NERVOUS
pruritis	Skin hypersensitivity resulting in severe local itching. SKIN, NERVOUS, CIRCULATORY, GLANDULAR
psoriasis	Persisting skin disorder, resulting in pink-reddish patches covered with whitish scaling. SKIN, GLANDULAR, CIRCULATORY
purpura	Abnormal blood hemorrhage into skin, mucous membranes, or body tissues, resulting in purplish patches of discoloraction.

CIRCULATORY, <u>SKIN</u>/<u>MEM-</u>
<u>BRANOUS</u>, <u>GLANDULAR</u>

radiation exposure,
radiotoxemia

<u>SKIN</u>/<u>MUSCULAR</u>, <u>GLAN-</u>
<u>DULAR</u>, CIRCULATORY

rash

General reddish eruption on
the skin, usually temporary and
associated with communicable
diseases.
<u>SKIN</u>, <u>GLANDULAR</u>, CIR-
CULATORY, NERVOUS

ringworm, tinea

Contagious and itching fungus
disorder of the skin, resulting
in vesicles and scales formed
into ring-shaped patches.
<u>SKIN</u>, <u>GLANDULAR</u>

rosacea

Sebsaceous disorder mostly
on the nose, face, and chin, resulting in papules, pustules,
and excessive tissue growth.
<u>SKIN</u>, <u>GLANDULAR</u>, CIR-
CULATORY

scabies, itch

Infectious skin disorder resulting in eczema eruptions and
intense itching.
<u>SKIN</u>, <u>GLANDULAR</u>

scalp problems

<u>SKIN</u>, <u>GLANDULAR</u>,
CIRCULATORY

sclerema, scleroderma

Hardening of the skin.
<u>GLANDULAR</u>, <u>SKIN</u>, CIR-
CULATORY, URINARY/IN-
TESTINAL

scratch
Superficial skin injury produced by scraping from fingernails, claws, or a rough surface.
<u>SKIN</u>, CIRCULATORY

sebaceous gland problems
<u>SKIN</u>, <u>GLANDULAR</u>, CIRCULATORY

seborrhea
Abnormal excessive secretion of sebum.
<u>GLANDULAR</u>, SKIN, NERVOUS, CIRCULATORY

shingles, herpes zoster
Inflammatory disorder along the spinal nerves, resulting in vesicular eruptions and pain.
<u>NERVOUS</u>, <u>GLANDULAR</u>, SKIN, CIRCULATORY

shiver(s)
Skin tremor from cold or fear.
<u>CIRCULATORY</u>, <u>NERVOUS</u>, <u>GLANDULAR</u>

sinus problem
<u>MEMBRANOUS</u>, <u>GLANDULAR</u>, CIRCULATORY

sinusitis
Sinus inflammation.
<u>MEMBRANOUS</u>, <u>GLANDULAR</u>, CIRCULATORY

skin problems
<u>SKIN</u>, <u>GLANDULAR</u>, CIRCULATORY, NERVOUS, URINARY/INTESTINAL

sore(s)
Local ruptured, abraded, or ulcerated tissues of the skin that is tender and painful.
<u>SKIN/MUSCULAR</u>, CIRCU-

stomatitis Mouth inflammation.
MEMBRANOUS/MUSCU-
LAR, <u>DIGESTIVE</u>, <u>GLAN-
DULAR</u>, CIRCULATORY

synovial problems <u>MEMBRANOUS</u>, <u>GLAN—
DULAR</u>, CIRCULATORY

thrush (see aptha, stomatitis)

tinea Any fungus disorder of the skin.
<u>SKIN</u>, <u>GLANDULAR</u>, CIR-
CULATORY

trachoma Chronic contagious conjunctivitis.
<u>GLANDULAR</u>, <u>MEMBRAN-
OUS</u>, CIRCULATORY

ulcer(s) Open sore or break in the skin
or membranous tissue, result-
ing in degeneration and often
pus formation.
<u>SKIN</u>/<u>MEMBRANOUS</u>, CIR-
CULATORY, NERVOUS,
GLANDULAR

**urticaria, hives, nettle
rash** Vascular reaction (allergy) of
skin resulting in raised, itching,
swollen areas on the skin or
membranes.
<u>GLANDULAR</u>, <u>NERVOUS</u>,
<u>DIGESTIVE</u>, CIRCULATORY,
SKIN

Vincent's angina, trench mouth

Contagious painful disease, resulting in ulceration of the mucous membrane of the mouth and adjacent parts.
MEMBRANOUS/MUSCULAR, GLANDULAR, CIRCULATORY, NERVOUS

wart

Skin protrusion or projection.
GLANDULAR, SKIN

wound

Break or cut in skin/membranous tissue caused by external violence.
SKIN/MEMBRANOUS, GLANDULAR, CIRCULATORY, NERVOUS

yeast infection problems

MEMBRANOUS, GLANDULAR, CIRCULATORY

CHAPTER THIRTEEN

HERBAL AID FOR CLEANSING/ SUPPORTING THE MUSCULAR AND SKELETAL SYSTEMS

Creative expression with body movement requires strength and flexibility

The muscular and skeletal systems (comprising muscles and connective tissues, bones and cartilage, and the like) are responsible for body support and expression. These important systems determine body form and also your capability for physical action. Healthy bones supply your body with strength, protection, and support, while your muscles serve as levers for body alignment, movement, and power. The muscular/ skeletal systems are interrelated in both composition and structure, and they require dynamic activity and regular relaxation for optimum performance.

Irritation, inflammation, and other degenerations of flesh and bone tissues relate to imbalances of excessive acid wastes and other impurities, or elemental deficiencies in the body. Particularly, these systems require minerals (such as calcium, silicon, phosphorous, or sodium) which are found abundantly in fruits, whole grains, nuts, vegetables, and selected herbs and can be supplemented also from seawater and animal sources. Body imbalances which produce excessive acid wastes, and which are not extracted efficiently from the blood and lymph, will result in sodium losses and degenerations within the stomach walls and joints. Muscular/skeletal tissues can be cleansed and supported by using cleansing herbs internally in the form of (cool) teas and herb capsules taken with ample water. Cleansing herbs will support muscular/skeletal operations by—

(1) extracting metabolic wastes and impurities efficeintly from cells and tissues;

(2) firming and strengthening structural tissues for added capacity and tenacity;

(3) balancing metabolic and functional activities so that

optimum performance is realized;

(4) supplying mineral requirements so that physical potentials and capabilities can be achieved; and

(5) arresting degenerations, catalyzing restorations, and promoting rejuvenation within all body systems.

Externally, these cleansing herbs are valuable muscular/skeletal aids as compresses, liniments, oils, poultices, vapors, baths, packs, and so on (which are introduced in the <u>HELP YOURSELF</u>! textbook, Course 1).

Muscular tone and skeletal alignment are indispensable to efficient blood circulation and for enabling adequate distribution of life-giving nutrition. Circulation blockages and nervous stresses (such as difficulties in abdominal organs, lower extremities, and respiration) may be due to mechanical pressures from spinal displacements, or muscular deterioration and prolapsus. Adequate exercise (such as sports, jogging, swimming, slantboard, or exercisers), massage therapy, chiropractic adjustment or alignment, grass or sand walking, and footbaths are invaluable means for aiding muscular/skeletal vitality. The more distressing muscular/skeletal problems and malfunctions relate to glandular difficulties (for instance, emotional stresses can lead to adrenal secretions which concentrate body energies into muscular tensions; or, liver disturbances can lead to impurity build-up and imbalances in the blood that directly affect body nutrition and metabolism).

Besides vigorous activity, another important factor in muscular/skeletal health building is rest. Rest is not just inactivity; it encompasses a time and means for releasing body tensions. Rest is achieved when body energies return to equilibrium and balance. Rest enables body systems to unburden themselves and to harmonize their functions, which may be accomplished with a warm bath, a relaxing swim, a nature walk, rhythmic movement, or quieting music. Your body will achieve maximum capability and make minimum tensions when you enjoy your work and total environment. Your muscles and skeleton were designed to conserve and channel body energies into dynamic and creative expression!

Major characteristic of single herbs which supply muscular and skeletal aid

ALFALFA leaves
Medicago sativa

Valuable minerizer and nutrient restorer, with excellent absorptive capability

COMFREY root
Symphytum officinale

One of nature's greatest tissue builders; contains allantoin which promotes rapid cell production; especially rich in organic compounds of calcium, potassium, phosphorus, sodium

GOLDEN SEAL root
Hydrastis canadensis

Considered by many as a healing "cure-all"; expecially restorative to severe flesh and membrane conditions; valuable disinfectant and antiseptic properties

MARSHMALLOW root
Althaea officinalis

Powerful nutritive healing aid; rich in organic compounds of mucilage, starch, pectin, oxygen, calcium, and minerals; powerful restorer for serious degenerative conditions

SLIPPERY ELM innerbark
Ulmus fulva

Powerful soothing nutritive restorer; rich bland mucilage that has the nutritive value of oatmeal; neutralizes systemal acidity and counteracts tissue degenerations

BLACK WALNUT hulls, leaves
Juglans nigra

Important herbal restorer for glands and tissues (espcially for persisting chronic disorders)

146

IRISH MOSS plant *Chondrus crispus*	One of nature's greatest mineralizers from the sea; general body alkalinizer and tissue restorer
HORSETAIL or **SHAVEGRASS** herb *Equisetum arvense,* *E. hyemale*	Powerful tissue cleanser-restorer, with high silicon and calcium content, plus organic acid compounds that are needed to fix calcium
PLANTAIN leaves *Plantago major*	Powerful blood cleanser-restorer (special influence on lymphatics); tissue builder and soothing restorer
YELLOW DOCK root *Rumex crispus*	Excellent blood builder (rich in iron) and tissue cleanser-restorer; powerful glandular aid

Basic herbal recipes (combinations) for supplying muscular and skeletal aid

_____ comfrey root, marshmallow root, slippery elm bark, ginger root, wild yam root, lobelia herb, (golden seal root, yellow dock root, nettle leaves)

_____ comfrey root, golden seal root, slippery elm bark, aloe leaves, (ground ivy leaves, clove flowers)

_____ comfrey root, alfalfa herb, oat straw, Irish moss plant, horsetail or shavegrass herb, lobelia herb, (elecampane root, boneset herb, prickly ash bark)

_____ golden seal root, capsicum fruit, myrrh gum, (echinacea root, eucalyptus leaves, elecampane root, clove flowers)

_____ comfrey root, white oak bark, mullein leaves, black walnut hulls, marshmallow root, gravel root root, wormwood herb, lobelia herb, scullcap herb, (sanicle herb, echinacea root)

_____ Siberian ginseng rootbark, Ho Shou-Wu root, black walnut hulls, licorice root, gentian root, comfrey root, fennel seed, bee pollen, bayberry rootbark, myrrh gum, spearmint leaves, safflower flowers, eucalyptus leaves, lemongrass herb, capsicum fruit, (dandelion root, ginger root)

_____ comfrey root, horsetail or shavegrass herb, oat straw, lobelia herb, (marshmallow root, boneset herb, myrrh gum)

_____ golden seal root, black walnut hulls, marshmallow root, lobelia herb, plantain herb, bugleweed herb, (echinacea root, prickly ash bark, clove flowers)

_____ comfrey root, marshmallow root, lobelia herb, chickweed herb, mullein leaves, (golden seal root, Irish moss herb)

_____ comfrey root, marshmallow root, mullein leaves, slippery elm bark, lobelia herb, (golden seal root, myrrh gum, capsicum fruit)

Problems and malfunctions involving the muscular/skeletal system

abscess

Localized collection of pus resulting from disintegration or displacement of tissue and surrounded by inflamed tissue. MUSCULAR, GLANDULAR, CIRCULATORY

ache

Persisting pain, either dull or severe. NERVOUS, MUSCULAR, CIRCULATORY, GLANDULAR

acromegalia, acromegaly

Abnormal elongation and enlargement of bones and tissues of extemities and head (in middle-aged persons). SKELETON/MUSCULAR, GLANDULAR, DIGESTIVE

akinesia, acinesia

Partial or complete loss of muscular movement. MUSCULAR, NERVOUS, GLANDULAR, CIRCULATORY

Albers-Schoenberg disease, osteopetrosis

Abnormal calcification of bones, easily fractured.

149

SKELETAL, GLANDULAR

ankylosis

Abnormal immobility and fixation of a joint.
GLANDULAR, SKELETAL

arthritis

Inflammation of a joint, often accompanied by deformation.
GLANDULAR, SKELETAL/ MUSCULAR, CIRCULTORY, NERVOUS

arthrosclerosis

Hardening or stiffening of joints.
GLANDULAR, SKELETAL, CIRCULATORY

arthrosis

Degeneration of joint
GLANDULAR, SKELETAL

ataxia

Muscular incoordination.
MUSCULAR, NERVOUS, GLANDULAR

atony, debility

Lack of normal tone.
MUSCULAR, GLANDULAR, DIGESTIVE, CIRCULATORY, NERVOUS

atrophy

Wasting of a part due to nutritional deficiency.
CIRCULATORY, NERVOUS, GLANDULAR, MUSCULAR

bee sting

Venomous wound from barbed stinger of a bee.
MUSCULAR, (astringent),

boil, furuncle

Tissue inflammation of sub-layers of the skin, gland, or hair follicle.
MUSCULAR, GLANDULAR, CIRCULATORY

bone problems

SKELETAL, GLANDULAR, CIRCULATORY, DIGESTIVE

bruise, contusion

Injury causing rupture of small vessels and discoloration in the sub-skin tissues.
MUSCULAR, CIRCULATORY, NERVOUS

burn

Injury to tissue to excessive exposure to radiant energy.
SKIN/MUSCULAR, NERVOUS, CIRCULATORY, GLANDULAR

bursitis

Inflammation of a sac or cavity in connective tissue near joints shoulder, elbow, knee, bunion.
MUSCULAR, GLANDULAR, NERVOUS, CIRCULATORY

calcification

Deposit of calcium in body tissues.
MUSCULAR/SKELETAL, GLANDULAR, DIGESTIVE

cancer	Malignant tumor or growth. <u>GLANDULAR</u>, <u>MUSCULAR</u>
carbuncle	Inflammation of skin and deeper tissues, with pusy degeneration through several openings, accompanied by constitutional reactions. <u>MUSCULAR</u>, <u>GLANDULAR</u>, CIRCULATORY, NERVOUS
caries	Gradual degeneration and decay of a tooth or bone often accompanied by inflammation of surrounding tissue and eventual abscess formation. <u>SKELETAL</u>/<u>MUSCULAR</u>, CIRCULATORY, GLANDULAR
cartilage problems	<u>SKELETAL</u>, <u>GLANDULAR</u>, CIRCULATORY
chilblain, frostbite	Inflammation and swelling of fingers, toes, feet, caused by cold, damp weather. <u>CIRCULATORY</u>, MUSCULAR, GLANDULAR
chorea	Nervous disorder with muscular twitching. <u>NERVOUS</u>, MUSCULAR, GLANDULAR

connective tissue problems	SKELETAL, GLANDULAR, CIRCULATORY
contusion	Injury or bruise in which the skin is not broken. MUSCULAR, CIRCULATORY, NERVOUS, GLANDULAR
convulsion(s)	Sudden attack of violent involuntary muscular contractions. NERVOUS, MUSCULAR, CIRCULATORY, GLANDULAR
cramp(s)	Spasmodic, painful, and involuntary contraction of a muscle. NERVOUS, CIRCULATORY, MUSCULAR, GLANDULAR
cyst(s)	Closed sac with a membrane and contents, developing abnormally in a body cavity or structure due to obstruction of a duct, parasitic infection, and the like. GLANDULAR, MUSCULAR, CIRCULATORY
emaciation	Extreme loss of flesh, extreme thinness, wasting away to become very thin. DIGESTIVE, GLANDULAR, CIRCULATORY, MUSCULAR

fibroma

Mild fibrous, encapsulated, connective tissue tumor. GLANDULAR, MUSCULAR/SKELETAL, CIRCULATORY

finger problems

CIRCULATORY, MUSCULAR/SKELETAL, GLANDULAR, NERVOUS

fissure

Deep ulcer or crack-like sore. MUSCULAR, CIRCULATORY, GLANDULAR

flesh problems

SKIN/MUSCULAR, CIRCULATORY, GLANDULAR, NERVOUS

foot/feet problems

MUSCULAR/SKELETAL, CIRCULATORY, GLANDULAR, NERVOUS

foreign bodies (removal of)

Slivers, dirt, or other foreign material in skin tissues, eyes, nose, and so on, often causing inflammation and infection. MUSCULAR, CIRCULATORY, GLANDULAR

fracture

Break in a bone structure at the spot where force was applied. SKELETAL, CIRCULATORY, NERVOUS, GLANDULAR

furuncle, boil

Deep-seated infection of hair follicle or sebaceous glands, resulting in inflammatory swelling of the skin and under-

154

lying tissues, and degeneration/destruction of a central core of tissue that is ejected as pus discharge.
MUSCULAR, CIRCULATORY, GLANDULAR

gangrene

Deficiency or absence of blood supply to body tissue causing its local degeneration and death.
CIRCULATORY, MUSCULAR, NERVOUS, GLANDULAR

gingivitis

Inflammation of gums.
MUSCULAR, CIRCULATORY, GLANDULAR

glaucoma

Eye disorder due to excessive pressure within the eyeball that results in damage and degeneration of the optic nerve, causing a gradual loss of vision.
GLANDULAR, CIRCULATORY, NERVOUS, MUSCULAR

gout

Metabolic disorder indicating blood impurity (especially uric acid) and causing sharp, painful inflammation around body joints, usually starting in the knee or foot.
GLANDULAR, URINARY/INTESTINAL, CIRCULATORY, MUSCULAR, NERVOUS

growth(s)	Abnormal cell mutiplication, such as in a cyst or tumor. GLANDULAR, MUSCULAR
gum problems	MUSCULAR, CIRCULATORY, DIGESTIVE, GLANDULAR
healing problems (general)	MUSCULAR, GLANDULAR, CIRCULATORY, NERVOUS
hernia, rupture	Organ protrusion or projection through connective tissue or a cavity wall in which it is normally enclosed or sustained. MUSCULAR, GLANDULAR, CIRCULATORY
infection	Invasion of a part by microorganisms, resulting in contamination, inflammation, pain, and disordered function. MUSCULAR, GLANDULAR, CIRCULATORY, NERVOUS
inflammation, swelling	Tissue reaction to injury, with capillary dilation, swelling, pain, and so forth. MUSCULAR, CIRCULATORY, NERVOUS, GLANDULAR
injury	Damage to a body part. CIRCULATORY, MUSCU-

LAR, <u>NERVOUS</u>, GLAN-
DULAR

jerking Sudden, often involuntary, muscular movement.
<u>NERVOUS</u>, MUSCULAR, GLANDULAR

joint problems <u>SKELETAL</u>, <u>GLANDULAR</u>, CIRCULATORY, URINARY

knee problems <u>SKELETAL/MUSCULAR</u>, CIRCULATORY, GLANDU-LAR, NERVOUS

leg problems <u>CIRCULATORY</u>, <u>MUSCU-LAR/SKELETAL</u>, <u>NER-VOUS</u>, <u>GLANDULAR</u>

leprosy, Hansen's disease Chronic contagious disease with enlarging, spreading no-dules and macules that para-lyze nerves, weaken muscles, with degeneration or deformity.
<u>GLANDULAR</u>, <u>MUSCU-LAR</u>, NERVES, CIRCULA-TORY

lesion(s) Abnormal structural change in an area or patch of tissue.
<u>MUSCULAR</u>, <u>GLANDULAR</u>, CIRCULATORY, NERVOUS

ligament problems <u>MUSCULAR/SKELETAL</u>, CIRCULATORY, GLANDU-LAR

lockjaw, tetanus Jaw muscle spasm and result-

157

ing inability to open the jaws.
NERVOUS, MUSCULAR, CIRCULATORY, GLANDULAR

lumbago

Dull aching pain in the loins or lumbar region.
INTESTINAL, CIRCULATORY, GLANDULAR, MUSCULAR, NERVOUS

marrow problems

SKELETAL, GLANDULAR, CIRCULATORY

motor problems

NERVOUS, CIRCULATORY, MUSCULAR, GLANDULAR

mouth problems

MUSCULAR, CIRCULATORY, GLANDULAR

muscular rheumatism

Abnormal muscular condition, resulting in inflammation, soreness, pain and local spasms.
MUSCULAR, GLANDULAR, CIRCULATORY, NERVOUS

muscle/muscular problems

MUSCULAR, CIRCULATORY, NERVOUS, GLANDULAR, DIGESTIVE, URINARY/INTESTINAL

necrosis

Localized death of areas of tissue or bones which are surrounded by healthy parts.
CIRCULATORY, MUSCULAR/SKELETAL, GLANDULAR, NERVOUS

158

nipple problems	MUSCULAR, CIRCULA-TORY, GLANDULAR
osteomalacia	Degenrative softening of bone structures, resulting in brittle-ness and deformitites, mostly in adults and women. SKELETAL, GLANDULAR, CIRCULATORY, NERVOUS, DIGESTIVE
obesity, adiposity, corpulence	Condition of excessive fat on the body, 20-30 percent over normal weight. GLANDULAR, MUSCULAR, CIRCULATORY, DIGES-TIVE, NERVOUS
opthalmia	Severe eye inflammation, usually from infection. MUSCULAR, CIRCULA-TORY, GLANDULAR, NER-VOUS
osteoporosis	Structural degeneration of bone, resulting in increased porosity through calcium ab-sorption. SKELETAL, GLANDULAR, CIRCULATORY, DIGES-TIVE
osteitis	Bone inflammation, often resulting in deformation. GLANDULAR, SKELETAL, URINARY/INTESTINAL
Paget's disease	Chronic inflammation of bone

with progressive degeneration and deformity (bending of long bones).
<u>SKELETAL</u>, <u>GLANDULAR</u>, CIRCULATORY, DIGESTIVE, URINARY/INTESTINAL

palsy

Paralysis condition resulting in sensory or motor discontrol, especially manifest as an uncontrollable tremor of the body or a part.
<u>NERVOUS, MUSCULAR,</u> GLANDULAR, CIRCULATORY

Parkinson's disease

Nervous degeneration resulting in a very fine and spreading tremor, progressive muscular weakness and rigidity, forward-bending posture and fast characteristic gait.
<u>NERVOUS, MUSCULAR,</u> CIRCULATORY, GLANDULAR

podalgia

Pain in the feet.
<u>NERVOUS</u>, <u>CIRCULATORY</u>, MUSCULAR, GLANDULAR

porosis

(See osteoporosis)

posture problems

<u>SKELETAL</u>/<u>MUSCULAR</u>, <u>GLANDULAR</u>, NERVOUS, CIRCULATORY

Pott's disease

Infectious inflammation of the

spinal vertabrae, resulting in bone destruction and curvature of the spine and often compression of the spinal cord and nerves.
SKELETAL, NERVOUS, CIRCULATORY, GLANDULAR

prolapsus

Falling or downward displacement of a body part or organ.
MUSCULAR, CIRCULATORY, GLANDULAR

pus

Yellowish-white fluid matter, resulting from inflammation and composed of albuminous substances, leukocytes, tissue debris, and the like.
MUSCULAR, CIRCULATORY, GLANDULAR

pyorrhea

Inflammatory and pusy degeneration of teeth sockets, resulting in loosing of teeth and gum recesssion.
MUSCULAR, GLANDULAR, CIRCULATORY, DIGESTIVE

rheumatic fever

Inflammatory, feverish and painful systemic disorder in and around the joints, and also resulting in inflammation of heart muscles and valves.
GLANDULAR, MUSCULAR/ SKELETAL, CIRCULATORY, NERVOUS

rheumatism

Various abnormal conditions of muscular soreness and stiffness, pain in joints and associated structures.
MUSCULAR/SKELETAL, GLANDULAR, CIRCULATORY, NERVOUS, URINARY

rheumatoid arthritis

Progessive inflammation and swelling of joints and cartilage, and pain.
GLANDULAR/URINARY, SKELETAL, CIRCULATORY, NERVOUS

sarcoma

Cancerous condition arising from muscular, bony or connective tissue.
GLANDULAR, MUSCULAR/SKELETAL, CIRCULATORY, URINARY/INTESTINAL

scurvy

Deficiency disease caused by insufficient vitamin C, resulting in spongy gums, teeth looseness, hemorrhaging or bleeding, abnormal bone formation.
MUSCULAR, GLANDULAR, CIRCULATORY, DIGESTIVE

skeletal problems

SKELETAL, GLANDULAR, CIRCULATORY, DIGESTIVE, URINARY/INTESTINAL

spasm

Sudden involuntary or convulsive muscular contraction.

162

NERVOUS, MUSCULAR, CIRCULATORY, GLANDULAR

spider bite
Insect with poisonous fangs
MUSCULAR (astringents), NERVOUS, GLANDULAR

spine/spinal (vertebrae) problems
SKELETAL, GLANDULAR, CIRCULATORY, NERVOUS

spondylitis
Inflammation of the vertebrae.
SKELETAL, GLANDULAR, CIRCULATORY, URINARY

sprain
Severe stretching or tearing of ligaments due to a violent twisting of a joint.
SKELETAL/MUSCULAR, CIRCULATORY, NERVOUS

stenosis, stricture
Narrowing or stricture of a passageway or orifice.
MUSCULAR, CIRCULATORY, NERVOUS, GLANDULAR

sting
Wound made by an insect, having a poisonous or irritating reaction.
MUSCUALR (astringents), NERVOUS, GLANDULAR

strabismus
Imbalanced coordination of eye muscles.
MUSCULAR, NERVOUS, GLANDULAR, CIRCULATORY

suppuration	(see pus)
swelling	Abnormal enlargement of a body surface. <u>MUSCULAR</u>, CIRCULATORY, GLANDULAR
teeth/tooth problems	<u>SKELETAL</u>/MUSCULAR, GLANDULAR, CIRCULATORY, NERVOUS
tetanus	Infectious disorder resulting in a persisting and painful spasmodic contraction of a voluntary muscle, especially the jaw. <u>NERVOUS</u>, <u>MUSCULAR</u>, CIRCULATORY, GLANDULAR
tetany	Intermittent nervous spasms of muscles in body extremities, associated with mineral deficiencies and parathyroid disorder. GLANDULAR, <u>NERVOUS</u>, CIRCULATORY, MUSCULAR
tic, twitching	Spasmodic muscular contraction, often associated with tension, involving facial and other muscles. <u>NERVOUS</u>, <u>MUSCULAR</u>, GLANDULAR, CIRCULATORY
tumor	Abnormal enlargement resulting in a new growth of tissue. GLANDULAR, <u>MUSCULAR</u>

164

ulitis   (see gingivitis)

undulant fever   Infectious disease with fever, weakness, pain, and swelling joints.
CIRCULATORY/<u>SUDORI-FEROUS</u>, <u>SKELETAL</u>, <u>GLANDULAR</u>, DIGESTIVE

whitlow, felon   Pus-forming inflammation at the end of a finger or toe.
<u>MUSCULAR</u>, <u>GLANDULAR</u>, CIRCULATORY, NERVOUS

wryneck, torticollis   Abnormal muscle contraction in neck resulting in drawing the head and chin toward a side position.
<u>MUSCULAR</u>, <u>NERVOUS</u>, GLANDULAR, CIRCULATORY

Selected Bibliography

Culbreth, David M.R., Ph. G., M.D. *A Manual of Materia Medica and Pharmacology.* Philadelpha: Lea & Febriger, 1927.

Font Quer, Dr. P. *Plantas Medicinales, El Dioscorides Renovado.* Barcelona, Spain: Editorial Labor, S.A., 1962.

Grieve, Mrs. M. *A Modern Herbal* (Vols. 1 & 2), New York: Dover Publications, (1931) 1971.

Holvey, David N., M.D., editor. *The Merck Manual of Diagnosis and Therapy,* Twelfth Edition. Rahway, N.J.: Merck Sharp & Dohme Research Laboratory, 1972.

Hutchens, Alma R. *Indian Herbology of North America.* Kumbakonam, S. India: Homeo House Press, 1969.

Kloss, Jethro. *Back to Eden.* Coalmont, Tennessee: Longview Publishing, 1939.

Millet, Edward Milo. *Help Yourself!* (Course 1 in Herbal Health-Building). Provo, Utah: The Institute of Creative and Natural Studies, 1978.

Millet, Edward Milo. *Improving Your Diet With Herbs/ Making Herb Therapy Easy.* Provo, Utah: The Institute of Creative and Natural Studies, 1976.

Nowell, Dr. Herbert. *Post Graduate Course.* Vancouver, B.C.: Dominican Herbal College, 1926.

Shook, Edward E., D.C., N.D. *An Advanced Treatise of Herbs* (mimeograph) and *Elementary Course in Herbology* (mimeograph). n.d.

Thomas, Clayton L., M.D., M.P.H. editor. *Taber's Cyclopedic Medical Dictionary.* Philadelphia: F.A. Davis Company, 1973.

Vander, Dr. Adrian. *Plantas Medicinales.* Barcelona, Spain: Ediciones Adrian Vander Put, 1970.

Wren, R.C. *Potter's New Cyclopaedia of Medicinal Herbs and Preparations.* New York: Harper Colophon Books, 1972.

HERB DICTIONARY (English-Spanish)

agrimony - agrimonia
alfalfa - alfalfa
angelica - angelica
balm - melia, tornjil
barberry - agracejo
bayberry - malagueta
birch - abedul, alamo blanco
bistort - bistorta
bittersweet - dulcamara
black cohosh - cimifuga
black walnut - nogal negro
bladderwrack - vejigoso, fugo
vejigoso, sargazo
blessed thistle, holy thistle -
cardo bendito, cardo santo
blue cohosh - hierba de San
Cristobal
boneset - eupatorio
buckbean - trebol de agua
buckthorn - palo de banon
bugleweed - licipo
burdock - bardana, lampazo
cactus - cactus
capsicum, cayenne - pimiento
cascara sagrada - cascara
sagrada
catnip - hierba gatera, nebeda
celery - apio
centaury - centaurea
chamomile - manzanilla
chickweed - pamplina, alsine
cleavers - amor de hortelano
cloves - clavo de especia
coltsfoot - farfara
comfrey - consuelda

coriander - cilantro, culantro,
coriandro
cornsilk - barba de maiz
couchgrass - grama de norte
Culver's root - veronica
damiana - damiana
dandelion - diente de leon
echinacea - equinacea
elder - sauco
elecampane - enula, helenio
eucalyptus - eucalipto
eyebright - eyfrasia
fennel - hinoho
fenugreek - fenofreco
garlic - ajo
ginger - jengibre
ginseng, Siberian - gensin
siberiano
golden seal - sello de oro, hidra-
stide de canada
goldenrod - vara de oro
gotu kola - gotukola
ground ivy - hiedra terrestre
hawthorne - espino
Ho Shou-Wu - Ho Shou-Wu
hops - supulo
horehound - marrubio
horseradish - rubano rustico
horsetail, shavegrass - equiseto
hyssop - hisopo
Irish moss - musgo de Irlanda
juniper - enebro
kelp - encina del mar
lady's slipper - chapin de venus,
cipripedio
licorice - regaliz, paloluz

linden - tilo
lobelia - lobelia, tobaco indio
lungwort - pulmonaria
marigold - maravilla, mercadela
marshmallow - malvavisco
mistletoe - muerdage
motherwort - agripalma
mullein - verbasco, gordolobo
myrrh - mirra
nettle - ortiga
papaya - papaya
parsley - perejil
pasque flower - pulsatilla
passion flower - pasionaria, pasiflora
peach - duraznero
pennyroyal - poleo
peppermint - menta
plantain - llanten
pleurisy root - raiz de asclepias
prickly ash - espino cerval
psyllium - psyllium
pumpkin - calabacera
red clover - trebol rojo
red raspberry - frambueso
rhubarb - ruibarbo
rosehips - cinarrodon
rosemary - romero
rue - ruda
safflower - alazor
sage - salvia
sarsaparilla - zarzaparrilla
saw palmetto - palmito enano
scullcap - esculetaria, terciananaria
senega snakeroot - poligala
shepherd's purse - bolsa de pastor

Siberian ginseng - ginsen siberiano
slippery elm - olmo americano
St. Johnswort - hierba de San Juan, hiperico
tansy - tanaceto
thyme - tomillo
uva ursi, bearberry - gayuba
valerian, garden heliotrope - valeriana, hierba del gato
vervain - verbena
violet - violeta
Virginia snakeroot - serpentaria
watercress - berro
white oak - roble blanco
white pond lily - nenufar blanco
wild lettuce - lechuga del monte, lechuga silvestre, serrallon
wood betony - betonica
wormwood - ajenjo
yarrow - milenrama, milefolio
yellow dock - acedera
yucca - yuca

Viscum album, 33
vitality, 15
  (defined), 15
  achieving greater physical, 19
  good circulation is essential
    for optimum, 19

W

WATERCRESS herb, 104
WHITE OAK bark, 130
wholeness and balance, 17
WILD LETTUCE herb, 34
WILD YAM root, 88
WITCH HAZEL leaves, bark, 130
WOOD BETONY leaves, 33
WORMWOOD herb, 95

Y

YARROW herb, 50, 61, 82
YELLOW DOCK root 103, 147
YUCCA root, 104
Yucca glauca, 104

Z

Zea mays, 61
Zingiber officinale, 83, 87

atony 150
atrophy 150
autotoxemia 122
autotoxication 110
autotoxicosis 122

B

bad breath 55
baldness 132
bedsore 132
bee sting 150
belching 89
biliousness 110
bedwetting 63
bite 132
bladder problems 63
bleeding 24
blister 132
blood (purity)
  problems 24
blood pressure (high) 24
blood pressure (low) 24
blood sugar, low 114
body odor 133
boil 151, 154
bone problems 151
bowel problems 122
brain problems 35
breast problems 73
breath problems
  (bad) 55
breathing problems 53
Bright's disease 63
bronchial problems 53
bronchitis 53
bruise 151
burn 151
bursitis 151

C

cachexia 110
caffeinism 97
calcification 151
calculus/calculi 63
callus 133
cancer 152
canker 133
carbuncle 152
carcinoma (see
  cancer) 152
cardiovascular
  problems 24
caries 152
cartilage problems 152
cataract 133
celiac disease 122
cell metabolism
  problems 110
cellulitis 109, 133
cephalalgia 36
cerebral problems 36
chafing 133
chest problems 53
chickenpox 86, 134
chilblain 152
childbirth problems 73, 75
chill(s) 24
chlorosis 73
choking 53
cholera 110
chorea 152
circulation
  problems 24
cirrhosis 110
claustrophobia 36
cleansing (to
  facilitate) 134

dyspnea 54
dysuria 64

E
ear problems 112
earache 42
eczema 135
edema 64
elephantiasis 135
elimination problems 124
emaciation 153
embolism 25
embryo development 74
emesis 99
emotion/emotional
  problems 112
emphysema 54
empyema 55
encephalitis 37
endocrine problems 112
endurance problems 112
energy problems 25
enteritis 124
enuresis 63, 64
enzyme problems 112
epidemic diseases
  (see communi-
  cable disease) 83
epidermis 135
epilepsy 37
equilibrium problems 37
erection problems 74
eruptive diseases 83
erysipelas 135
erythema 136
estrogen deficiency 74
evacuation problems 124
excretion problems 124

exhaustion 25
eye problems 136

F
face problems 136
fat problems 112
fatigue 25
fear 38
female problems 74
feminism 74
fever 83
fever blister 136
fibroma 154
finger problems 154
first aid (herbal) 25
fissure 154
fit 38
flatulence 90
flesh problems 154
flu 55
food poisoning 97
foot/feet problems 154
foreign bodies
  (removal) 154
fracture 154
frigidity 74
frostbite 136, 152
frustration 38
furuncle 151, 154

G
gallbladder problems 113
gallstone 113
gangrene 155
gas 90
gastric problems 90
gastralgia 90
gastritis 90

joint problems 157

thymus problems 117
thyroid problems 117
tic 164
tinea 142
tobacco habit 42
tonsil problems 58
tonsillitis 58
toxemia 117
trachoma 142
tremor 47
trench mouth 143
tuberculosis 58
tumor 164
twitching 164
typhoid fever 85
typhus fever 86

U
ulcer(s) 142
ulitis 165
undulant fever 165
uremia 66
ureteritis 66
urethritis (see pro-
    state problems) 78
urinary/urine
    problems 66
urticaria 142
uteritis 79
uterus/uterine
    problems 79

V
vaginal problems 79
vaginismus 80
vaginitis 80
varicella 86

varicose veins 29
variocele 79
variola 85
vascular problems 30
vein / venous
    problems 30
venereal disease 79
vertigo 37
Vincent's angina 143
vitality problems 30
voice/vocal problems 58
vomiting 99
von Reclinghausen's
    disease 47

W
wart 143
whitlow 165
whooping cough 56
worm problems 125
wound 143
wryneck 165

Y
yellow fever 84
yeast infection
    problems 143